and Health Care

Carol Spengler, R.N., M.S.

Director, Department of Nursing
Mid-Missouri Mental Health Center
Columbia, Missouri

Womanpower and Health Care

Copyright © 1976 by Marlene Grissum and
Carol Spengler

First Edition

Library of Congress Catalog Card No. 75-41571

ISBN 0-316-32895-2

Printed in the United States of America

This book is dedicated to our mothers,
who gave us love and understanding,
and to our families and special friends,
who continue to sustain that love

Preface

This book represents our efforts to focus on some of the special issues, problems, and barriers confronting women, particularly nurses. At first, our major support and inspiration came from each other. We shared an interest in and concern for women, especially those who happen to be nurses, and spent hours over a long period of time heatedly discussing injustices to women in general and nurses in particular. As our awareness of these injustices grew, our anger increased also. Eventually we were able to direct our energy toward more constructive activities and to begin formulating our ideas for this book.

Out of our variety of work experiences we each formulated ideas and concepts of what nursing practice is and what it could be. Many of the concepts that eventually found their way into the book were a result of those experiences. We talked with many of our colleagues when we traveled around the country to attend meetings and workshops, and it was noteworthy to us that many reported similar problems in their work settings and shared common concerns. Thus we learned that the problems and concerns we were focusing on are national in their scope.

Other issues and problems concerning women were viewed from two very divergent life-styles. It was both amazing and reassuring for us to discover that our perspectives regarding the major issues were similar even though one of us comes from a very large family, is married and a mother, and the other is single, has no children, and grew up in a small family.

The first section of this book is devoted to the idea that the socialization process of childhood leads women to be passive, dependent and indecisive. We explore some of the attitudes and behaviors of both men and women that help to perpetuate an outmoded role for women in this society and illustrate that the socialization process makes it extremely difficult for female nurses to become autonomous practitioners who have the ability to make independent decisions concerning nursing practice.

The second section demonstrates that women — and nurses — can break out of the traditional mold that holds us in the past. We explore the concepts and theories of change and the willingness or unwillingness of women to be change agents and risk-takers.

Once women begin to understand the socialization process, it is easy for them to grasp the difficulties in initiating change or becoming a risk-taker. Change is an integral part of our society. How women accept it and learn to use the strategies connected with it will, in great measure, determine their sense of self-esteem, their power and their control over their own lives.

The issues discussed in this book are emotional and political, but we believe they can be resolved in a constructive and rational manner. Awareness of the specific problem areas must be developed, however. Coupled with this awareness, an understanding must be gained of how the indoctrination of women perpetuates characteristic modes of behavior that prevent women from sharing a more significant and powerful role in such a major social institution as the health care system.

M. G.
C. S.

Acknowledgments

From the beginning we were fortunate to have a great deal of support from some very special people. They helped us immensely in a variety of ways, and we want to express our thanks.

We are especially grateful to Inge Mauksch, because it was while working on a project with her that we became acquainted and eventually decided to write this book together. Her enthusiasm and interest in our progress were very encouraging. She also introduced us to Christopher Campbell of Little, Brown and Company, who believed in our capabilities when we were very doubtful. He and all the staff at Little, Brown were extremely pleasant and helpful while we were completing the manuscript.

Throughout the writing of this book, many women became interested in our project and provided various kinds of support. We want to extend special thanks to them: to Judith Schultz for enlightened discussions and books loaned; to Susan Wood for providing resource materials; to Mary Steiner, Rhonda Anson, and Trudy Gardner for supplying us with information and reading materials from the Behavioral Sciences Library of the University of Missouri; to Ginny Volmert, Barb Harnar and Barb Roby for typing early drafts of the manuscript (usually under great pressure); to Mary Love and Janis Holzhauser for their special kind of encouragement and support; and to Arthola Brown, Pat Richards, Audrey Hurley, Patsy Lowe, Brenda Closser, Marlyn Richards, Rosann Wisman, Judy Atterberry and Shirley Keyes, who provided understanding and support in the work situation. Once we committed ourselves to writing this book, we automatically involved those individuals who are closest to us, and they were especially supportive. Indeed we wish to thank them. The Grissum family took on some new and added responsibilities but managed to sustain and support us with love and understanding. So to Clyde, who became both mother and father, and to Terry, Cynthia and Beth, we acknowledge our gratitude. And a special thank you to Jackie, who gave many hours to a variety of tasks as well as to reading and criticizing parts of the manuscript. Meanwhile, in the other household, the total environment was converted into the authors' retreat until the book was finished, and everyone adapted their life-style a bit. A very special man, Bob

Spengler, played an important role in helping us as we worked on this project. He was our friend in the true sense of the word. He not only encouraged us but provided constructive criticism of the manuscript, supplied us with helpful resource materials, saw that the coffeepot was always full and kept us well nourished with generous home-cooked meals. Pat MacRae was quietly supportive and magnanimous in allowing us to take over her space in the household with a myriad of books, papers, and similar materials.

Gail Benjamin and Fannie Lu Davis are two special friends who were very helpful to us in critiquing sections of the manuscript. This was time-consuming for them but very beneficial to us. They were supportive and enthusiastic and gave us the boost we needed when we were hesitant or doubtful at times about our progress.

We are very appreciative of the interest and assistance that Larry Hill provided us. We are grateful for his generosity in lending his publishing expertise in relation to various aspects of the manuscript.

We are especially indebted to Virginia Wharton and to Nancy Megley of Little, Brown and Company for their invaluable assistance in editing this book.

Contents

Womanpower and Health Care

1 Conditioning of the Female

Carol Spengler

The women of today are in a fair way to dethrone the myth of femininity; they are beginning to affirm their independence in concrete ways; but they do not easily succeed in living completely the life of a human being. Reared by women within a feminine world, their normal destiny is marriage, which still means practically subordination to man; for masculine prestige is far from extinction, resting still upon solid economic and social foundations [1].

Simone de Beauvoir

to Her Role in Life

Numerous books on sale today provide in-depth and detailed analyses of the "socialization" process to which women are subjected in American society. In this book, we will attempt to summarize some concepts about women and to compare what happens to women in society as a whole with what happens to women in the smaller society of the health care system.

For centuries, we have continued to socialize children in rigid sexist roles. When they behave in a culturally defined way, we then attribute this to nature. Some of us have even gone so far as to attribute these behavioral differences between boys and girls to genetic or biological factors. The fact that sound scientific research has not proved this does little to discourage us from accepting it as truth.

More important, in each culture it has been the men who have defined "normal" female behavior. Men have also been expected to function in specific roles, but again, it has been the men who defined their own roles. The result has been a concentration of power in men. This fact undoubtedly accounts for the minor role

2   assigned to women throughout recorded history. "Socialization is the process by which the child learns to interact with the expectations and obligations of various groups. Essentially it is learning and living the culture of the group to which one belongs" [2].

The differences between males and females cannot be overlooked, but are the differences any more than biological? A woman, like a man, is a human being. Each is a unique, separate individual having a rich variety of potential for developing into a creative, productive being.

As all of us, men and women, are molded, shaped and formed to function in specific roles within the society in which we live, a comparison of the numerous factors that contribute to our molding and socialization will help to clarify the position of contemporary women.

As individuals, we develop within a specific social setting. We learn to perceive as required by our culture. Each culture and, at least to some extent, each group that an individual belongs to expresses a set of expectations and relationships. These influence the eventual development of attitudes, behaviors and social skills [3]. We know that over time these expectations and relationships do change or vary in some ways as people, social conditions and economic conditions change. One of the most consistently unchanging of these, however, is the role or position of women. Virtually every society has formed a set of implicit and explicit rules for proper behavior based on sexual differences [4]. Although the plight of the female has improved with time, the world today is still divided by the sexes — this is a man's world, and in it the woman has her place [4].

"Anthropologists, sociologists, theologians, prophets, seers, shamans and witch doctors interpret the web of ideas we have woven in an endless number of ways, but none is more central to the life of the individual or more vital to society than the patterns of behavior constructed around the physical facts of sex differences" [5]. Each generation changes slightly in its thinking about these sex differences. The factor that does remain constant, however, is that societies continue to ascribe different psychological attributes to men and women and on this basis to assign different duties and modes of living to each sex. It is *assumed* that societies do this

because the sexes have different intellectual, moral, social and
physical capabilities [6]. These assumptions have been adhered
to even though they have been disproved, so it may be asked why
they are perpetuated with each new generation. Elizabeth Janeway
has concluded that society has to assert as fact a social mythology
that it "depends on to cushion, to manipulate and – above all –
to explain the onrush of events, the demanding present, the im-
minent and frightening future" [7]. In order to elevate and equalize
the role and position of women today, we must first identify those
attributes and differences assigned to women which serve to perpetuate and reinforce the mythology about women.

Women and Their Stereotypic Roles

To begin with, women in our society are made out to be stereotypes.
It is asserted by psychologists, psychiatrists and some educators
that a woman's primary motivation in life, based on her true nature,
is to become a companion to a man and to become a mother [8].
A woman is defined in terms of a man rather than as an independent
being. (Interestingly, a man is never defined in terms of a woman.)
A woman, moreover, is expected to show ability in attracting men.
If she is successful in this, she will acquire a home. She can then
begin to carry out her alleged major mission in life – that of fulfilling
her natural and nurturing role of wife and mother [9]. The role
of wife and mother is an important one. It is extremely satisfying
and rewarding to many women. It is restrictive, however, to assert
that this is the major role for all women. For some, it would be
stifling. When women do not choose the role of wife and mother as
a life-style or when they choose to combine marriage with a career,
it is implied that they are failing to adjust to the normal female
nature.

In her book *The Second Sex*, Simone de Beauvoir retraces the
historical evolution of the role and position of women from the time
of the early nomads, through the early agricultural communities,
through the Middle Ages and up to the present time. Throughout
this evolutionary process, she illustrates the primacy of the male.
At no time has woman ever imposed her own law – her place in
society has always been the one that men have assigned to her. At
times, woman was fortunate in being more deeply integrated into

society. When this occurred, she shared a significant role with her
male companion and played a prominent role in history [10]. Her
liberty, however, was empty, because she remained as always the
property of the master — man [11].

From century to century, woman has assumed the major role
in child care. Along with this nurturing aspect of her role, woman's
work has mainly been associated with food-gathering and preparation,
clothing manufacture, crafts and maintenance of the home [12].
This is still true today. Even when women work outside the home
and share in the domestic economy of the family, they enjoy fewer
social and economic privileges and they live a much more difficult
life than their husbands: whether she is a farm wife, a business
woman, a professional woman or a worker employed in any of a
number of jobs outside the home, woman still remains responsible
for the care of the children and the maintenance of the household
[13]. For the woman who seeks to combine a career and motherhood, there is another difficulty — her masculine competitors occupy
most of the interesting and advantageous positions. This is partially
because her skills are less specialized. She has often not had the
same educational opportunities. Also, discrimination based on sex
has been an effective barrier for many women in the job market.
All too frequently, although she has the same skill and knowledge
and carries out the same tasks, she will not receive the same pay as
a man in the same position. The Bureau of Labor Statistics recently
published the results of area wage surveys covering six industry
divisions; the results indicated that, on a nationwide basis, pay
levels were consistently higher for men than for women working
in the same occupation [14].

The majority of books our children are using in schools continue
to depict women primarily in the role of the wife and mother who
remains in the home to care for the family. Television commercials
and programs, newspaper and magazine advertisements, along with
other aspects of industry, continue to promote the major role of
women as consumer and housewife. This is despite the fact that
statistics indicate otherwise. The recordbreaking growth achieved
by American industry since 1940 was, in part, made possible by
the phenomenal increase in the proportion and number of women,
especially married women, who joined the work force [15]. Women
now constitute over 40 percent of the work force in nonagricultural

industries in America. Of that total number, 60 percent are married.
Of those who are married, 30 percent are mothers with children
under the age of six years [15].

For the past 30 years, the service industry has ranked first in
the employment of women. It is interesting to note that many of
the jobs in the service industry have been described as extensions
of what women do at home as homemakers — such as teaching
children and young adults, preparing food and nursing the sick [15].

From 1940 to 1970, men shifted into better paying, more prestigious professional-technical jobs. In the education field, male
teachers in colleges and universities make up 70 percent of the
faculty. In elementary and high schools, 70 percent of the teachers
are women. Law, medicine, engineering and many other professional-technical fields have remained significantly male dominated
[16].

Besides the nurturing characteristics attributed and relegated to
women alone, other stereotypes are assumed. Women are characterized as emotionally unstable, weak, intuitive, inconsistent,
dependent, passive, empathetic, sensitive, subjective and interpersonally oriented [17, 18]. The image that is usually presented
of the male in our society is in direct contrast: he is characterized
as aggressive, independent, competitive, task-oriented, stoic, analytical, rational, self-disciplined, confident, able in leadership, objective,
emotionally controlled and outward-oriented [18]. While some of
the characteristics attributed to women are positive, most are viewed
as negative in our society. The traits attributed to men, on the
other hand, are strongly valued in American society. Again, the
educational system, the communications media, the business industry and the major social institutions, along with psychiatrists
and psychologists, perpetuate the feminine stereotypes. Aside from
the fact that some basic biological differences have been identified
between males and females and explain the difference in some physical
functioning, only minimal scientific evidence has been presented by
psychology and psychiatry to explain behavioral differences between
the sexes [19]. In the meantime, "evidence is accumulating that
what a person does and who he believes himself to be will in general
be a function of what people around him expect him to be, and what
the overall situation in which he is acting implies that he is" [19].

It is an accepted practice among scientists not to promote a theory

6   as valid until it has been tested and confirmed [20]. Freud and many others who have advanced theories about women and the female nature have not met even the most basic conditions of a scientific approach [20] — yet their theories have been accepted and applied as valid. What other factors contribute to the traditional stereotyping of women? Why does society continue to define women in less positive and less powerful roles than men? Why are social myths perpetuated?

These queries could be explained in part by what Christine Pierce calls the appeal to the "natural." She states that "for centuries people have appealed to the 'natural' to back up their moral and social recommendations" [21]. She stresses that it is difficult for anyone in any moral or social context to say what he means by "natural." She notes further that usually what is argued as natural is defined as "good" [22], which implies that the opposite of "natural" is usually abnormal or bad [23]. Many of the characteristics mentioned earlier in connection with women are considered "naturally" feminine. For example, it is "natural" for women to have children and to remain in the home to care for them. It is a woman's "nature" to be nurturing, sensitive, empathetic and interpersonally oriented. Many women, however, have these qualities in varying degrees. Also, there are women who either lack these qualities altogether or have them to a much lesser degree — and yet, they are functionally competent in many ways. Are these women to be considered abnormal or unnatural? On the other hand, some men are nurturing, sensitive, empathetic and interpersonally oriented. By many standards, men with these qualities have often been defined as womanlike or effeminate. Such characteristics, however, have little to do with biological sex differences. We develop these traits because we have the capacity as human beings to show our caring and concern for others through our behavior, i.e., nurturing, sensitive, and empathetic behavior directed toward others. We *all* have the potential to develop these characteristics regardless of our gender.

Many consider a woman unnatural and unfeminine if she is aggressive, logical, analytical, rational, and independent. Yet it can be a pleasure to know and work with the many women who have these characteristics. However, since they do not fit the norm, they are sometimes considered a threat to other women and definitely a threat to men.

It is our society as well as civilization as a whole that produces the creature known as woman [24]. In our American society, children are "socialized" to grow up and become men and women who will be like society's ideal norm. "Socialization refers to the pressures — rewarding, punishing, ignoring and anticipating — that push the child toward evoking acceptable responses" [25].

Human beings are social beings — and their interactions with other people are what make them distinctly human. Because of this, it is difficult and at times inappropriate to draw conclusions about human behavior that are based on research with animals. Yet, this is a common practice. All children, regardless of their cultural group, have the same basic needs. The way in which children are taught to manage their needs differs depending on the society in which they exist. All of us, as children, were expected to learn behaviors that are consistent with and appropriate to a particular societal standard [2]. Children, from the time they are young infants, have behavioral tendencies that parents and other individuals who are close to them respond to. These tendencies are determined by the adults' own individual values as well as widespread social values related to acceptable child behavior [25].

It is recognized that there are behavioral differences between boys and girls in infancy and early childhood. For example, girls display less overt physical aggression, are less active physically, are more sensitive to physical pain, display greater verbal, perceptual and cognitive skills and have significantly less genital sexuality than boys. Boys, on the other hand, are prone to act out aggression, have higher activity levels, are more physically impulsive, are genitally sexual earlier and appear to have less well developed cognitive and perceptive skills than girls [25]. "Girls' characteristic behavior tends to disturb parents less than boys' characteristic behavior. The perceptual, cognitive, and verbal skills which for unknown reasons are more characteristic of girls enable them to analyze and anticipate adult demands and to conform their behavior to adult expectations" [25]. This can be interpreted that girls would be in a better position to cope with the world than boys if the socialization demands were the same for both sexes [25]. While these behavioral differences in young children are important, the responses that adults make to these tendencies probably account for many sex differences in adults.

Little girls appear to have an advantage over boys early in life because many characteristic responses are acceptable for them but are prohibited in boys. For example, it is not acceptable for a boy to be too aggressive or too passive. A girl's behavior, however, is permitted to range from ultrafeminine to athletic tomboy. Even more important, dependent behavior, which is normal for all young children, is permitted in girls (and probably encouraged) but is not tolerated in boys [26]. "Thus, girls are not encouraged to give up old techniques of relating to adults and using others to define their identity, to manipulate the physical world and to supply their emotional needs. Girls' self-esteem remains dependent upon other people's acceptance and love; they continue to use the skills of others instead of evolving their own" [26]. On the other hand, boys at an early age learn to develop a sense of self and criteria of worth fairly independent from the responses of others. "A boy turns to achievements in the outer and real world and begins to value himself for real achievements in terms of objective criteria" [26]. Boys have a more difficult early childhood in that they are pressured to give up their childish ways and to begin to *earn* their masculinity. These childish behaviors are considered "feminine" and acceptable in girls; they do not have to be earned [27]. It is easy to see that in the long run, girls do not have the real advantage because their socialization results in delaying their search for identity and development of autonomy and internal criteria for self-esteem. Girls become conformists, and this affects what happens to them in the adult world.

It is easy to see that behavioral sex differences observed in infancy and early childhood are enlarged through the socialization process [27]. For example, aggressive behavior displayed by boys is encouraged and therefore reinforced by adults because they believe that boys should behave this way. Aggressive behavior in girls is discouraged because it is considered inappropriate. As adults, then, when men are aggressive and women act in a more gentle, less assertive way, these behaviors are considered predetermined and therefore natural characteristics of each sex; the fact that they are promoted and reinforced is not recognized.

Boys and girls up to about the age of 12 years are comparably strong in both mental and physical powers. The little girl, however, is indoctrinated with her vocation in life from her earliest years [28]. Since the major responsibility for child care rests with the mother in a family, it is she who will provide most of the direction and reinforcement in shaping the child into her "natural" feminine role. The father supports the socialization process by assuming a protective attitude toward his daughter, thereby reinforcing her passive, dependent nature. Many others close to the child get in on the act of socializing her — aunts, uncles, grandparents, neighbors, teachers — and all these people reinforce those traits considered to be *naturally* feminine. Little girls are reminded frequently through a variety of means that girls perform specific tasks and behave in specific ways. For example, "little girls are mama's helper." They are then encouraged to help mama around the house and are given toys to play with that are similar to mama's tools and utensils. Through their play and their toys, girls are assisted in identifying with their mother. This will ultimately prepare them for their "natural" role in the adult world. If their brother shows an interest in such things, he is told he is a "sissy"; such things are only for girls. If a little girl shows an interest in mechanical or other pursuits that have been designated masculine, she is reminded that only boys or men perform such activities. If she persists in showing an interest in such pursuits, she will be pressured into giving these up. Comments are made such as "It's not ladylike or feminine to do that." Most of us have succumbed to those whispers in our ears, and we behave as female adults — just as we have been programmed to behave.

Very young children at play exemplify this theory. At an early age, both little boys and girls are active and inquisitive. All children love to climb, to explore, to discover new things. Little girls are as mischievous and brave as little boys are. Little boys are as loving and gentle as little girls are. It is then that the "whispers" from the significant people in their lives begin to turn into "shouts and screams." Eventually, both boys and girls learn to play the game and to develop their "natural" roles.

A personal example illustrates my point. I was the only daughter, reared with a brother slightly older and one slightly younger. My brothers were taught from an early age that they should "protect" me and never hit me because I was a girl. Except on a few rare occasions, both of my brothers followed those guidelines (much to their exasperation, and eventually to mine). I learned very early that I could verbally antagonize them until their fists were clenched in anger and the blood vessels stood out on their necks, but I never had to fear their retaliation. When the situation sometimes grew too intense and they would threaten to throttle me, I would run to my mother and tell her. She would then remind them that they were not to hit me because I was a girl.

At that time in my life, I felt that it was a distinct advantage to be a girl. As we grew older, my brothers as well as other members of my family were careful to protect me in many different ways, and this too I perceived as a definite advantage. When my rights were impinged upon for one reason or another, there was always someone stronger than I who would willingly fight my battles, and I remained a passive but grateful observer. As a young child, I laughed at my luck in not having to suffer the disadvantages of my brothers. As a young woman, however, I learned slowly and pain-fully the protection by others interfered with my development as a self-confident, self-directing individual. Being passive and protected was actually a distinct disadvantage. I also learned that it takes a great deal of time and effort to unlearn such conditioned behavior — perhaps an entire lifetime. In our society, much human potential and creativity are wasted in this manner — especially in the case of women.

There are definitely biological necessities for both sexes. Women bear children and nurse them. There are many aspects of the nur-turing process, however, that could be carried out by men (and is in some work roles) if men were socialized and expected to do this. "It is easy to confuse statistical predominance with norm, and to explain norms as being 'only natural'" [29]. An explanation that is convincing is not based on normative generalizations or desires but rather on specific facts. This then provides a logically consistent and empirically complete reasoning for cultural and sexual differences [29].

It is a commonly accepted fact that behavior that is rewarded is reinforced. We need to turn our attention to the rewards in the socialization process. Both boys and girls are rewarded for behavior that is considered appropriate to their sexuality. As previously pointed out, women are the primary socializers of both sexes, since child care is chiefly their responsibility. For a boy, this means then that he is trained to be a male by a female. He learns to be a boy not by identifying with his teacher (mother) but by acting in a manner that she tells him is "manly" [30]. The mother respects the boy's maleness. The boy has an advantage in that his mode of existence in relation to other people eventually leads him to assert his subjective freedom [31]. "His apprenticeship for life consists in free movement toward the outside world; he contends in hardihood and independence with other boys, he scorns girls" [31]. He is active and explores; he participates in rough-and-tumble games; he is proud of his strength and proud of his sexuality; he learns to scorn pain and to hold back tears; he is bold and daring; and he learns to test and challenge his own manhood [31]. "It is by *doing* that he creates his existence, both in one and the same action" [32]. A boy reared in our society usually has many options to choose from; depending on his own innate capabilities and motivations, he has a fairly good chance to achieve success (as defined by American standards). Aggressiveness and independence on the playground are considered important characteristics to be fostered because they will help prepare the boy for his role in society as a "normal" male. He will be reminded over and over, by parents and others, "a man doesn't cry," "a big boy doesn't play with dolls," "only girls take care of babies," etc. When he feels pain, he will be encouraged to be stoic. He will receive approval from adults by becoming independent of them [33]. Very early, boys are persuaded that more is demanded of them because they are superior. This is to give them courage for the difficult path that they will have to follow [33]. Growing up masculine must be a heavy responsibility for little boys, but the rewards for it are very great.

In all societies, the pursuits of men are considered to be the most prestigious; on the other hand, the activities of women are devalued [34]. If child care were the primary responsibility of men in our country, there would surely be more value and importance given to it. Many men and women believe that only men are able to do the "important" things that contribute to society, such as exercising political power, being creative and artistic, and playing an important role in the economy [34]. Is it any wonder that a boy is seldom heard to claim that he would rather be a girl. He would be unwise to consider it when it is still very obvious that he is living in a "man's world" in which women occupy only a minor place. On the other hand, it is not at all uncommon to hear a girl exclaim that she wishes she were a boy. Freud would have labeled this "penis envy." I would call it merely an astute observation about the real world, showing the girl's desire to be part of it.

The socialization process for girls is quite a contrast to that for boys. A boy's maleness is respected by the mother. This allows eventually for greater independence and autonomy. She fully plans to fit her daughter into the feminine world, however [35]. "The daughter is for the mother at once her double and another person, the mother is at once overweeningly affectionate and hostile toward her daughter; *she saddles her child with her own destiny:* a way of proudly laying claim to her own femininity and also a way of revenging herself for it" [35]. The girl's apprenticeship for life is not one of free movement like her brother's. Instead, she begins her socialization with a conflict. The conflict is between her existence as an autonomous person and as an object who exists to please others [32]. Since one of her main goals in life will be the latter, she will have to make herself a passive object and therefore renounce her autonomy. "She is treated like a live doll and is refused liberty" [32]. She is not encouraged, as the boy is, to be assertive and independent; to develop her strengths and then to be proud of her achievements; to be bold and daring in both work and play. Instead, the mother spends a great deal of time shaping the girl in her own image to ensure that she develops into a "true woman" [35]. Since children spend the greatest amount of their time with their mothers, there are abundant opportunities for little girls to see and learn their "natural" feminine roles. Not only have most of us been taught how to cook, sew, clean house, shop for groceries and do laundry and other household chores, but we were taught many other feminine virtues and wiles that will help us to become better wives and mothers.

Goals of Women

As stated earlier, to become a wife and mother is still the ultimate goal of the majority of women in our society. This is not surprising when the overt and covert pressures brought to bear on the young woman are considered, how she is trained to fit into the established norm and to be content with this. Boys are also socialized toward marriage; however, there is an important difference. "No young man considers marriage as his fundamental project" [36]. Ask a boy or young man what he wants to do in the future and he will usually mention an occupation or special interest. Ask a girl or young woman the same question and she will still frequently say "I want to get married" as though she considers this an occupation. Even if she does mention a true occupation, it is usually "until I get married." This clearly illustrates how effective feminine socialization is.

From a fairly early age, girls are discouraged from being noisy, overactive, and competitive in games or sports (if they insist on participating in such things). Then they are taught to choose clothes that reflect the latest styles but which frequently have nothing to do with comfort, to apply makeup properly and to carry themselves gracefully – all mostly to please men. While careful grooming can certainly add to the attractiveness of an individual, it has made many women prisoners in their own bodies.

At the same time that young girls are being socialized into traditionally feminine roles and personality, they are also being taught how to achieve academic success in school. Both boys and girls are rewarded for such achievement in their early schooling. Interestingly, until puberty, girls actually excel academically. It seems that until girls reach puberty, those who are academically successful have evolved a " 'bisexual' or dual self-concept" [37]. Both boys and girls are permitted to compete in academic areas. When the girl is rewarded for this type of success, she "evolves a self-concept associated with being able to successfully cope and compete" [37]. At puberty, however, the requirements of femininity and "normalcy" change and move closer to the stereotype for female adulthood. At this time, then, femininity for girls, like masculinity for boys, becomes an attribute that must be *earned* [37]. On the one hand, the girl has been taught and rewarded for success. Then, at a specific time period in her life, all those pressures that reinforced her academic achievement now work to enforce her preparation for the traditional female role. Success now entails becoming a good wife and mother, and only this. This paradox makes it quite clear to girls that their traditional female role and all the values that go with it are less desirable, less valuable in the progress of humanity and the world [38].

It seems abundantly clear that, except in unusual circumstances, women in American society merely serve as appendages to men.

14   True, there have been a very few great women scientists, artists, poets, explorers, musicians, politicians, etc., a fact that illustrates how sadly we have wasted the talents and potential of over half of our human population. It is interesting to speculate on what the future would hold if women were socialized differently. If they were given the encouragement, opportunity, support and reinforcement that their brothers have known for so long, they could doubtless make the most of their true potential if they chose to do so. The very notion that girls are *taught* by their mothers to be nurturing, passive and therefore "feminine" dispels the myth that these attributes are natural or part of woman's "nature." If mothers would spend as much time teaching their sons such characteristics, it seems reasonable to expect that, over time, most children — regardless of sex — would develop into adults with these attributes. At the same time, if mothers and fathers would encourage their daughters to become more independent, self-directing, adventuresome individuals who did not find it necessary to live their lives through others, we would find many more autonomous, self-actualized women.

Early socialization affects the female throughout her life. It influences her personality development and coping mechanisms as well as her choice of life-style and occupation. Whatever her lifestyle or her chosen work, she will be under the influence and control of men in one way or another. Factors that bear this out are examined and emphasized throughout this book. As succinctly stated by Simone de Beauvoir, it should be remembered that "the true control of the world has never been in the hands of women; they have not brought their influence to bear upon technique or economy, they have not made and unmade states, they have not discovered new worlds. Through them certain events have been set off, but the women have been pretexts rather than agents" [39].

References

1. de Beauvoir, Simone. *The Second Sex.* New York: Vintage Books, 1974, p. xxxv.
2. Dinkmeyer, Don. *Child Development — The Emerging Self.* Englewood Cliffs, N.J.: Prentice-Hall, 1965, p. 145.
3. Ibid., p. 144.
4. Janeway, Elizabeth. *Man's World, Woman's Place: A Study in Social Mythology.* New York: Dell, 1971, p. 7.

5. Ibid., p. 8.

6. Ibid., p. 9.

7. Ibid., p. 10.

8. Weisstein, Naomi. Psychology Constructs the Female. In *Woman in Sexist Society: Studies in Power and Powerlessness*, Gornick, Vivian, and Moran, Barbara (Eds.). New York: Basic Books, 1971, p. 207.

9. Ibid., p. 208.

10. de Beauvoir, op. cit., p. 105.

11. Ibid., p. 109.

12. Chodorow, Nancy. Being and Doing: A Cross Cultural Examination of the Socialization of Males and Females. In *Woman in Sexist Society: Studies in Power and Powerlessness*, Gornick, Vivian, and Moran, Barbara (Eds.). New York: Basic Books, 1971, p. 261.

13. de Beauvoir, op. cit., pp. 151–152.

14. Waldman, Elizabeth, and McEaddy, Beverly J. Where Women Work: An Analysis by Industry and Occupation. *Monthly Labor Review*, U.S. Department of Labor, Bureau of Labor Statistics, May 1974, p. 11.

15. Ibid., p. 3.

16. Ibid., p. 7.

17. Weisstein, op. cit., p. 221.

18. Bardwick, Judith M., and Douvan, Elizabeth. Ambivalence – the Socialization of Women. In *Woman in Sexist Society: Studies in Power and Powerlessness*, Gornick, Vivian, and Moran, Barbara (Eds.). New York: Basic Books, 1971, p. 225.

19. Weisstein, op. cit., p. 210.

20. Ibid., p. 211.

21. Pierce, Christine. Natural Law Language and Women. In *Woman in Sexist Society: Studies in Power and Powerlessness*, Gornick, Vivian, and Moran, Barbara (Eds.). New York: Basic Books, 1971, p. 242.

22. Ibid., p. 243.

23. Ibid., p. 245.

24. de Beauvoir, op. cit., p. 301.

25. Bardwick, op. cit., p. 226.

26. Bardwick, op. cit., p. 227.

27. Ibid., p. 228.

28. de Beauvoir, op. cit., p. 302.

29. Chodorow, op. cit., p. 269.

30. Ibid., p. 273.

31. de Beauvoir, op. cit., p. 315.

32. Ibid., p. 316.

33. Ibid., p. 305.

34. Chodorow, op. cit., p. 275.

35. de Beauvoir, op. cit., p. 317.

36. Ibid., p. 482.

37. Bardwick, op. cit., p. 229.

38. Chodorow, op. cit., p. 282.

39. de Beauvoir, op. cit., p. 147.

2 The Indoctrination

Carol Spengler

It is impossible for nursing to achieve real professionalization and lower the drastic drop-out rate among our practitioners, or for us to assume control over ourselves as individuals and as a collectivity, to take more active roles as innovators and instigators of social change, and to develop a career-orientation until we have elevated the position of all women — and of nurses [1].
Karen T. Lamb

# of Female Nurses

The health care industry is one of the biggest business enterprises in the United States, the total health expenditures in 1974 amounting to over 104 billion dollars [2]. This represented 7.7 percent of the country's Gross National Product, or a per capita expenditure of 485 dollars [2]. It is common knowledge that there is a crisis of almost overwhelming proportions in American health care. Because of the significant conquests we have made in various diseases, many people contend that we have one of the finest health care systems in the world. The system, however, has not been able to distribute services on an equal basis to those in need [3]. "If this system has failed to provide the kind of care that we would like, it is in large part because our population has grown enormously and in ways that foster increased demands for greater care. At the same time, we are still groping for the institutions, facilities, and personal resources that can meet the public's demands and match the advances that have come through medical research" [4]. Those consumers who have taken advantage of the services offered are now experiencing dissatisfaction and disappointment. The factors that

17

18 have brought about this dilemma in health care are multiple and complex. A great deal of in-depth study, evaluation and long-range planning will be required to correct the multiple problems within this gigantic and complex system. It is not the intent here to analyze the total health care system. Instead, only the parts of the system that relate to the profession of nursing will be examined.

"Nursing in particular holds the key to maintenance of humane, individualistic concern for people and their health problems" [4]. Our society is demanding changes in the health care delivery system that will meet contemporary needs. Nursing must, therefore, grasp the opportunity to play a greater, more significant role in effecting these changes. By analyzing and improving both nursing practice and nursing education, nursing professionals can improve the delivery of health care to the American people.

Nurses represent the single largest group of health care professionals in this country [5], numbering close to a million and a half. Nearly 800,000 of that number are employed in various health care settings [6]. Despite a slight increase in the number of men choosing nursing as a career, less than 2 percent of all nurses are males [7]. These statistics show that nursing is still primarily a "woman's" profession.* The special problems that are confronted by all women in our society are, of course, experienced by nurses as well. The characteristics, the concerns, the problems, the frustrations, the exploitations experienced by women everywhere can be easily seen in the everyday work world of the professional nurse. Just as women everywhere must become *aware* of the barriers in society that prevent them from developing their full potential, so must nurses. The conditioning of women and its effects on their role in life directly correlates with the conditioning of nurses and its effects on their traditional role in the health care setting. We cannot expect to improve the quality of nursing (and ultimately the quality of health care) or to expand the role of the nurse without first analyzing her role as a woman.

Nurses function in specific ways because of how they have been defined within the health care system. The role and place of the nurse in the total system correspond to the minor role assigned to women in American society as a whole. It is men who have assigned

*Henceforth in this book the word *nurse* will refer to the female nurse unless specifically stated otherwise.

this role to them, and many nurses themselves have accepted and perpetuated the situation, demonstrating the effectiveness of the programming and socialization process. The attitude of these nurses is considered "normal" because they have unquestioningly accepted the traditional role.

As stated previously, all individuals develop within a prescribed social setting, where they learn to perceive and behave as they are expected to in order to meet the norms of the group. When the young woman leaves her family and community subgroup to embark on a career in nursing, she joins a new culture that also has a set of prescriptions for proper behavior. She enters the world of nursing through a specialized educational program. Schools of nursing are the young woman's first exposure to this world. Her educational socialization wields tremendous influence on her behavior throughout her professional career. Consequently, many books and studies have been published regarding nursing education in this country. Because of the impact nursing education programs have on future practitioners, it is worthwhile to examine some of the usual characteristics and problems that prevail in those programs.

Nursing Education
To begin with, nursing education, whether in a hospital setting or a college or a university, is dominated by men. Hospitals are controlled by boards of trustees, hospital administrators and physicians; these are predominantly male. Colleges and universities are also male dominated (91 percent of all physicians, medical and osteopathic, 56 percent of all hospital administrators and 77 percent of all college administrators are males [8]). These are the individuals who control the budget, set the policies and manage the organization. In short, they control the system. This is not a surprising revelation; it merely corresponds to all other institutions within our society. It does, however, have an important bearing on nursing education. In a comprehensive study carried out by Lysaught on nursing and nursing education, a broad area of consensus was identified regarding the major problems of programs in nursing education. Three predominating difficulties were apparent: there is a shortage of qualified faculty; there is a lack of funds and adequate financing; and facilities are outmoded and inadequate [9]. That these conditions exist tells

us something about the way the public views nursing, the way those who control the health care system view nursing, the way politicians view nursing and, more serious, how nurses view nursing. If nursing were perceived as important and necessary, appropriate funding would be made available to help rectify this problem. Compare, for example, the type of support received by the medical profession in terms of space and money. The state and federal governments both contribute a significantly greater amount of money for medical education. The amount of support in the form of library facilities, office space, classrooms and economic fringe benefits are embarrassingly greater for medical schools.

One has only to tour an institution having both a medical school and a nursing school to observe the obvious discrimination. In many institutions, the medical schools have carpeted, brightly decorated and spacious private offices for their faculty, while the faculty of the school of nursing have offices that are small, colorless, carpetless and often shared by three or four faculty members — an indication of the nursing school's true importance. A visit to the library tells the story even more clearly. The vast majority of the books on the shelves are for the use of medical students. Of course, student nurses take advantage of them also. As for budgets, in many universities, schools of nursing are still under the direct or indirect control of the school of medicine. Even when they are autonomous, they are not viewed as such by school administrators [10]. Because of this, very often the budget for the school of nursing is added as a section under the medical school budget. When this occurs, the dean of the school of nursing is often in a position of having to justify expenditures to the dean of the medical school. Worse yet, she may have to virtually beg for a fair share for nursing education. Laboratory space and equipment in schools of nursing are commonly inadequate and inferior to the same facilities in the medical schools. The scarcity of modern, up-to-date equipment for nursing students is frequently a problem, and it points out what is truly valued in the system. There are schools of nursing in this country that do not have these problems, but they are in the minority. The nursing student does not have to be in the system very long before she notices all this. Her socialization into the nursing world has begun. She has now learned that the tools and the environment

necessary to prepare men for their work, medicine, are more valued
than the tools and environment needed to prepare women for their
work, nursing.

Program content and methods of teaching are important means
for preparing the student for her future role. Unfortunately, much
of nursing education today still resembles a military organization in
that orders are given and dutifully carried out [11]. When one reviews the historical development of our profession, beginning with
Florence Nightingale, we are painfully aware of how our subservience
began. It is totally inappropriate, however, a hundred years later,
to maintain a subservient and authoritarian approach to education.
Nursing should be in the mainstream of the contemporary social
scene if we are to help solve the problems that plague our nation.
We must prepare practitioners who can deal effectively with these
issues. To do this, students must be given the appropriate background
and preparation to become agents of change and leaders. They
must learn to use a scientific and systematic approach to the assessment and solution of human problems. They must be inquisitive,
creative and bold. Since much of their earlier life experiences and
socialization probably did not foster such behavior, it should be
encouraged in their professional education. Unfortunately, this
does not happen very frequently. To begin with, students do not
find enough adequate role models among their faculty [12]. What
they see usually are powerless, noninnovative faculty members who
conform to and perpetuate the feminine stereotype. They do this
through their behavior and their mode of communication with
students and also by educating students in outmoded, traditional
curricula that do not prepare them for the real work world. With
this type of traditional teaching, "we prepare a trained dependency
characterized by high predictability of behavior" [13]. The student
soon learns to play the game properly with her instructors to get
through the program. Students who are overly inquisitive or who
challenge their instructors are soon labeled troublemakers or poorly
suited for nursing. "In many institutions the nursing curriculum
seems to go out of its way to train conforming bureaucrats" [14].

Whether the student is labeled a conformer or a troublemaker,
she soon learns that a major part of her educational experience still
involves learning dates, doses, duties and procedures rather than
learning to pursue intellectual endeavors in a scholarly and scientific

fashion [15]. It is not that nursing curricula are lacking in the necessary background in the physical, social and behavioral sciences, liberal arts and humanities. Quite the contrary. Nursing education standards today are for the most part adequate in these areas and the educational process very rigorous. It is the application of knowledge acquired in these areas that creates a problem for students. They feel that they are hampered in using this knowledge in a creative way because they are expected to conform to the ideas of their teachers. Also, a great deal of classroom time is spent on irrelevant or unrelated material [15]. A personal example illustrates this point. Most of us spent some time in our program in a course dealing with the history and trends of nursing — but most of the focus was on history and there was very little on current trends. While we need to know where we came from, we also need to know where we are going, particularly as it relates to the larger society. One of the most important subjects that should be included in a course such as this is the history of women — not only in nursing but in health care, in other professions and in American society as a whole. Certainly, a study of the future of women would be pertinent because the history of nursing so closely parallels the history of women. To this day, there are nursing faculty members who see no reason to discuss the women's movement with their students or to include it in any course or seminar, as though this major social issue has no relevance to nursing. It is no wonder that the large majority of nurses graduate to enter the work world and never become involved in any controversial social issues. Their socialization from early childhood and throughout their professional education has been consistent: it has reinforced the traditional passive feminine role. Only the environment and subgroup have changed. The mother as chief socializer has been exchanged for their nursing instructor.

It would be easy merely to chastise our mothers and our nursing faculty for perpetuating and reinforcing the sexist, traditional roles by which we are hemmed in, but they are no more to blame than we are. Criticism serves no useful purpose, since we know that all of us have been programmed in much the same way. What we need to do instead is to break out of this vicious cycle and work toward developing a greater awareness of our potential as women. Certainly, a logical place to begin is with appropriate changes in nursing education. To do otherwise is inexcusable and irresponsible.

The most fundamental, important skill that nursing students today are being taught is the ability to provide effective care to individuals in a variety of settings. Most of the student's education is directed toward developing her future role as a professional practitioner. Historically, nursing has shared a prime role with medicine in providing care and treatment to patients. For a long time, the role of the physician has been well defined; the role of the nurse has been more ambiguous, and as a result, many people are confused. For example, the general public has a rather nonspecific view of the nurse; physicians, administrators and even some nurses have an occupational view of the nurse; however, an increasing number of nurses and other health care workers view nursing as an emerging and distinct profession different from medicine. All these views influence our expectations and the direction of nursing [16]. Traditionally the position of nurses has been one of implementing the purposes and programs of physicians in the area of medical care. Additionally, nurses have the potential to function autonomously in other areas of the health care spectrum [17]. Physicians are primarily concerned with curing illness or disability. "The central focus of nursing is care, comfort, guidance, and assisting individuals to cope with problems that lie along the health-illness continuum. It is the concept of the degree and nature of the deviation from a normal life process, or the degree and nature of deviation from a predictable psychologic or physiologic response to illness or disability, that distinguishes nursing practice from medical practice" [18]. The nursing student must learn those functions that she will carry out in her role as a practitioner. These functions include case-finding, diagnostic assessment, care supportive to life and well-being, health-teaching, individual or family health-counseling, therapeutic intervention (psychological or physiological) and restorative services [19]. Nursing by its very name and definition is a nurturing process. To be nurturing, to be caring, tender and compassionate, to be able intuitively to relate well with others, to be supportive of others' wants and needs — all are considered to be major feminine traits [20]. These traits most assuredly have been fostered and reinforced in women, and more specifically in nurses. A very pleasant, warm feeling is experienced when providing tender, compassionate care to someone who is in need of it. The ability to be nurturing, when it is appropriate and necessary, is probably

one of the most positive results of our early socialization as
women and nurses. It is unfortunate that the majority of men
in our society, because of their rigid and stereotyped socialization,
do not have the privilege of developing this trait also.

Although this is an attribute that women and nurses should
zealously retain, is it valued? Perhaps, by the individual who receives this type of care when it is needed. How does this service
compare to the type of service rendered by the physician? As
stated earlier, the physician primarily focuses on medical treatment and/or cure for a specific illness or disability. In order to
do this, he uses a variety of methods to reach a diagnosis of the
problem, and he then prescribes an appropriate treatment regimen.
Much of this treatment is carried out by others, including the nurse.
The physician's role and his functions could be primarily characterized as masculine in nature. He is expected to be decisive,
objective, persistent, rational, aggressive, courageous and dominant
[20]. This is not to say that all physicians are noncaring individuals.
Rather, the work that they do is considered to be in keeping with
accepted masculine behavior. Caring for the patient, a feminine
responsibility, is left to the nurse. Nursing care, to be effective,
must also be based on objective, rational and scientific principles
carried out in a decisive manner. Not many recognize this aspect
of nursing care. Further, they do not view the nurse as one who
functions in the same manner as the physician. The physician
usually spends a relatively short time with the patient, then leaves
the patient in order to do other work related to treatment or diagnosis. The nurse remains in close proximity to the patient for a
much longer period of time, in order to care for him. The physician's
role is very much like that of the father who is in the home only
part of the time and then leaves for work. The nurse (like the
mother) remains to care for the patient (the children). Because
of the organization of the health care system, the patient is put in
a dependent, childlike role. This simulated family situation is not
to the advantage of the patient or of the nurse.

The student nurse is in some ways spared the negative social
and/or parental pressures that other professional women students
must endure, because her work is accepted and viewed as an extension of what women should do — care for others. Women law
students, medical students, engineering students and the like are

tested more rigorously than their fellow classmates. They are also isolated from them more, are treated with deference and their femininity is questioned. I have talked with numerous women students in this position who repeatedly describe this as their experience.

Care and cure, then, are different, and yet both are important to the well-being of patients. In our present system, however, care and cure are not equally valued. To the idealistic and naive student nurse, this fact may not be apparent initially. Many experienced nurses may not have realized or accepted this fact either. How do we know it to be true? To begin with, there is an assumption that since much of nursing practice is concerned with caring for people, it requires primarily an intuitive process. Again, because it is considered to be a natural feminine attribute, it therefore requires very little knowledge or skill to carry out. We as nurses know this to be completely inaccurate. Human beings are complex. A great deal of scientific knowledge and skill are required to provide the kind of care that will effectively meet their needs, healthy or ill.

Some very obvious situations should indicate to the student that her nursing care is not highly valued. Her clinical experience will include care for the acutely ill patient, and an important part of her responsibility will be to assist the patient in his rehabilitation in order to ensure his return to maximal functioning. She is also responsible for helping him through health-teaching, to understand his illness. This will enable him to cope better with his rehabilitation. As part of her plan of action, she will work with him, his family or other individuals. She has been taught that the patient's recovery will be more successful if he has been properly prepared and informed; she has also been taught that it is the patient's right to expect this type of care and preparation. She may still be working closely with the patient at the time when the physician orders his discharge, for the physician may determine, without any previous discussion with the student or the nursing staff, that a cure of the acute aspect of the patient's medical condition has been effected or the condition has been controlled to the extent that he may now leave the hospital. The fact that the patient is still in need of "care" is not considered. The patient is then released from the hospital without the adequate information or preparation necessary for him and/or his family to deal with his aftercare. Many patients have been stripped of their dignity and independence upon entering the hospital system, and often they do not raise objections when their care is not as good as it should be. In fact, many patients are not even cognizant of their human rights as patients. To the student nurse, this is confusing and disappointing. As she sees a patient being discharged who she knows has not been adequately prepared, a conflict will frequently arise in her mind because she has been taught one thing but observes another. Worse, she knows that she is quite powerless because she is *only* a student nurse. She soon learns that when she attempts to solicit the support of her faculty and other nursing staff, they too are powerless to bring about a change in the decision.

Patients have been sent home with new colostomies that they have not been taught to care for; with drains and dressings in place that they did not know how to change; with newly diagnosed illnesses that require special diets or medication for adequate health maintenance, not understanding why they needed these or how to manage such a regimen; with prescriptions for medications with no explanation of how to take them or no means for purchasing them; and with a newly diagnosed medical or psychiatric condition that was briefly explained to them in medical terms that they did not understand but did not have the courage to admit. A talk with relatives, neighbors, or friends who have recently been hospitalized will bear this out, and it explains in part why the public is critical of health care today. The "care" component is devalued and in some ways almost nonexistent. On occasion, a patient's stay in a teaching hospital has been prolonged and extraordinary or complex tests have been ordered to enhance the learning experiences of medical students. Sometimes this has benefited the patient and sometimes not. One thing is certain: it cost either the patient or the taxpaying public more money. The advancement of knowledge or technology should not be discouraged, especially if it has the possibility of benefiting the patient; however, reevaluation regarding our priorities and our treatment of patients is long overdue.

Another frequent example of the low value placed on nursing care is this: A student or nurse may be providing some aspect of care to a patient when his physician or a group of physicians make rounds. The nursing care may be interrupted regardless of inconvenience to the patient, who may be indisposed at the time, and to the nurse. This type of situation not only devalues the nursing care being given but demeans the patient as well. All too often, we have excused this type of situation because we know that physicians are busy people. What is not considered is that the nurse is busy too! When interruptions like this occur, it is easy to see why she has difficulty organizing her time. Also, the patient should be considered in these situations. Often a patient has questions to ask his physician and looks forward to the opportunity to talk with him. When the doctor is on rounds in a group of strange physicians and the patient is receiving some form of treatment or care, however, it is hardly an appropriate time to attempt to communicate.

Another area that will demonstrate to the student that the skills she is developing are not highly valued is the type of ongoing research she will be exposed to. She will see that efforts are directed primarily toward research that will enhance knowledge about disease processes, about both preventive and curative medicine. She will rarely be exposed to scientific investigation directed toward increased knowledge or improved skill in providing nursing care. It would be very easy simply to criticize nurses, both practitioners and educators, for being remiss or disinterested in research, and it is true that many nurses lack concern or skill in conducting it. Once again, though, it should be pointed out that this results partially from their socialization. Research has not been established as an important priority in our profession until recently. The greatest contributing factor is, however, that nurses are not given the financial support or the necessary time to carry out much-needed research. Very little money has been appropriated to support the kind of research so desperately needed in nursing; again, nursing is merely women's work and not important enough, it would seem, to investigate. There are nurses who are very interested in conducting nursing research but are not given the necessary time away from their usual work to do it. In university settings, where it is expected that faculty will devote some time to research, writing and publishing, nursing faculty fall far short of their colleagues in other disciplines. Nursing faculty are distinctly different from other faculty because they usually have a much heavier schedule devoted to classroom teaching, clinical supervision and individual student conferences. Along with this, they have to prepare and grade assignments. All this leaves very little time or energy for research, writing and publication [21]. Very seldom are faculty members or practicing nurses hired for the sole purpose of conducting research. In both settings, there is a great need for well-qualified nurses either to teach or to give patient care; however, the supply is scarce. If there were enough individuals to fill those positions, the budget would probably not be adequate to support nursing research. This inequitable situation robs the student nurse of positive role models. It also robs her of an important body of knowledge that could contribute to the improved practice of nursing. Finally, it reinforces her image of nursing as a profession whose services are considered necessary but whose contributions to research are devalued.

Another major problem in nursing education that affects the socialization of future practitioners is the isolation that tends to characterize the schools. Baccalaureate and Associate Degree nursing programs located in colleges and universities share the isolation that is usually characteristic of medical schools, both often being located, and treated, separately from the main campus. In medicine this separateness pays off; in nursing it does not. The separateness of medical schools may be self imposed to obtain special economic privileges or to remain exempt from some general university policies. Also, medicine has a highly respected status within the university system, and its isolation has a different and more positive meaning than the separateness of the nursing school, which suffers the isolation without any of the accompanying advantages or status. For example, the nursing school may be located off campus in overcrowded and poorly equipped facilities without access to teaching tools available to other schools and students. Medical schools, on the other hand, though they may be located off campus, usually have more spacious, well-equipped facilities — often more impressive and costly than any other program. Nursing schools are "separate" to be sure — but definitely not "equal" [10].

In hospital schools of nursing, the isolation is even more complete. For the most part, the classrooms, faculty offices, laboratories and student housing are all in close proximity. Except for those courses taken on college campuses, the students and faculties are, in a sense, cloistered.

So — in both the university and hospital setting, the students and faculty experience physical and intellectual isolation from their peers. In this lonely position, both groups are often perceived by other faculty and students as inferior scholars in a second-rate discipline [10]. Those students in the various educational settings who either live away from the hospital or live in off-campus housing or in non-nursing dorms have a greater opportunity for interesting dialogue, exchange of ideas and social intermingling with fellow students or friends from varying backgrounds [10]. This does enhance their development of a broader perspective regarding life in general. It may also increase the students' ability to communicate with those other than nurses. It can assist them in cultivating relationships with individuals from other disciplines as well. This would be a beneficial outcome, since all disciplines, as well as the lay public, must learn to work together and respect one another if the delivery of health care services is to be improved. Nursing faculty and students must become a part of the hospital or university mainstream. It is to the advantage of both groups to do so as expeditiously as possible; otherwise, they will remain the stepchild of both groups.

When a young woman enters the world of nursing, she begins her initial socialization into the profession through an established educational program. In numerous ways, her education reinforces the socialization process she has experienced from early childhood. The meek will graduate and function as professionals in the stereotypic image of the majority of women in other walks of life. They will be submissive and conforming. They will be dependent and lack real autonomy. They will probably provide adequate nurturing care to their patients. They will never be in the vanguard, however, when overdue constructive changes are brought about in the nursing profession. Their wasted talent and untapped potential will be sadly missed when other nurses organize collectively to strengthen and elevate their role and position in the health care system. A large share of the responsibility for the development of these individuals rests within our own profession. Many of our schools have perpetuated society's myths about the attributes and roles of women.

The Lysaught study reported that "approximately one out of three entering students in nursing withdraws before graduation. This figure varies somewhat among institutions, and within geographic areas, but remains a relatively constant diminution factor" [22]. Many studies and investigations have been carried out to determine what factors account for these high attrition rates. Unfortunately, no reliable measurements have been developed, and therefore no specific reasons for this problem have been identified [22]. It may be that some who left did so because they were disillusioned and could not play the traditional feminine role. Did they feel stifled and inhibited by their nursing socialization? No one has the answer to this question. It is a matter for concern, however, and I hope that someday there will be specific answers. It could have far-reaching effects on our profession. More importantly, it could help us to evaluate our educational socialization process.

Across the country, there are some progressive faculties who have instituted innovative changes in their curricula; however, these programs are still in the minority. The idea that nursing education needs to be radically restructured is not new. The question is, how, in what direction and when will we restructure the system? Until we determine this, we will continue to perpetuate the sexist, powerless role of nurses through a major socializing system — nursing education.

The Real Work World

When the student graduates and joins the thousands of other nurses in the health care system, the main focus is on providing "illness" care as opposed to prevention and health maintenance. Because of this, hospitals (as opposed to some other types of institutions) continue to be predominant employers of professional nurses. The latest available figures indicate that nearly 65 percent of all nurses employed are working in hospitals. The second largest employers of nurses are nursing homes, with almost 7 percent actively employed. The remainder work in public health (including schools), nursing education, occupational health and private-duty nursing [6]. Regardless of the work setting, nurses find that they have many common problems. The work setting, like the educational setting and the community setting, constitutes a social subgroup. Again, prescribed behaviors that conform to established standards within the particular social system are promoted and reinforced. The graduate nurse enters the social system as a new professional who still has intact a great deal of her idealism about health care. When she moves from the student role to the professional role, she begins to enlarge her perspective of the health care system and her role in it. Many new individuals will share in socializing her further. To begin with, her peers, because of their close, working relationship, will serve as role models. They may also be a source of support by helping her to adjust to her new role with its incumbent responsibilities. She will be influenced to a great degree by their attitudes and their methods of functioning as they care for patients. All this can be positive or negative. Her response and adjustment depend mostly on her own motivation, capabilities and attributes, to be sure. Her education, past experiences and socialization will also influence her to a great degree.

Role and Scope of Nursing Practice

The role and scope of nursing are quite diversified and promise to become even more so in the future. In order better to understand the problems of nursing practice, a definition of its scope must be arrived at. One of the most comprehensive and meaningful definitions was made as a result of the Lysaught study. A logical representation was constructed on the basis of the following data: an extensive review of literature in the health field that included critical evaluation of more than 900 reports on the utilization of nurses and related personnel involved in providing patient care; over 100 on-site visits throughout America, including surveys and related interviews; personal observations made in all types of employment settings for nurses, such as hospitals, industrial plants, clinics, public health agencies and educational institutions; and discussions with over 1,000 nurses, physicians, administrators, students, consumers and researchers. On the basis of the findings in all these areas, a conceptual model was developed to illustrate the variables in nursing practice [23]. Nursing was then described "on the basis of a three-dimensional figure — a cube that permits us to assign spatial entity to practice while simultaneously considering three key variables" [24]. The three variables are: specific *nursing behaviors;* the *condition of the patient;* and the *environ-*

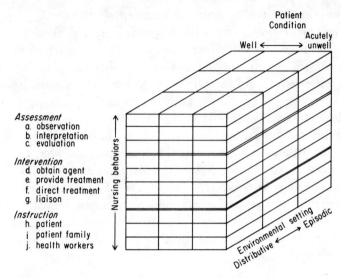

Figure 1 Interactive model of three variables in nursing practice: nursing behaviors, patient condition, and environmental setting. (From *An Abstract for Action, National Commission for the Study of Nursing and Nursing Education,* by Jerome P. Lysaught. Copyright © 1970 by McGraw-Hill Book Company. Used with permission of McGraw-Hill Book Company.)

mental setting in which care is given [25]. Figure 1 illustrates the relationships between the variables.

In the category of *nursing behaviors,* the primary tasks of nurses are subdivided into assessment, intervention and instruction. These activities, as carried out by nurses today, entail both simple and highly complex functions. Unfortunately, neither the public nor many other health care workers realize or understand this fact. For example, in the area of assessment, the observation process includes such traditional tasks as taking vital signs. More complex observation skills include taking a patient history, monitoring cardiac changes and performing a complete examination of the physical and/or mental status. When the nurse translates inferences about patient care into concrete action, "interpretation" has taken place as part of the assessment process. Assessing the results of treatment, auditing patient responses and identifying priorities for care are all aspects of the evaluation process used by nurses [25].

In the area of intervention, the primary nursing activities are broadly subdivided into the following: obtain agent, provide treatment, direct treatment and act as a liaison. Again, the tasks carried out in any of these areas may range from simple to complex. Examples of some very basic tasks might be as simple as calling a physician, making a bed or discussing a patient with another health care worker. A more dramatic example of intervention is when the nurse initiates cardiopulmonary resuscitation or defibrillation. This kind of action by the nurse requires errorless judgment and performance and is a matter of life or death for the patient [25]. The nurse has considerable responsibility in coordinating the treatment plan established by a multidisciplinary team of health care workers. Many of the activities carried out by the nurse in the course of a day can be identified as liaison activities. The nurse, as compared to other health care professionals, is usually closest to the patient. As a result, she has the task of communicating information, questions and/or plans to others. (This aspect of the role will be dealt with later in more depth.)

In the last area, instruction, the scope and quality of the nurse's educative role have continually enlarged. Instruction ranges from teaching classes to expectant parents to specialized teaching in relation to various aspects of rehabilitation for specific illnesses. Not only is the nurse responsible for teaching patients with regard to health and illness, but she is also involved in teaching the family and/or others significant in their lives. The pediatric nurse practitioner provides a good example of the nurse's educative role. She may work primarily with children who are healthy. As she works with them, she also teaches the parents about health maintenance in order to keep the child healthy. The nurse working in an ambulatory care setting may primarily see patients with chronic or debilitating illnesses. Since these patients are not healthy but may be only mildly ill, her teaching role will focus on the specific needs of this type of patient [26]. Regardless of the type of setting or the type of patient she is caring for, the nurse will always have a vital role in health-teaching. As we begin to focus more on primary prevention and health maintenance, the nurse will play an even greater role in health-teaching.

A significant aspect of the nurse's role as an educator involves other health care workers. In most health care settings, an important group of workers are employed to assist the nurse in providing care to patients. These individuals are classified as allied nursing personnel and comprise two distinct occupational groups: licensed practical nurses and assistants to nurses. The latter group consists of nurses' aides, orderlies, nursing assistants, attendants and home health aides [27]. Most of these individuals receive their initial education in an established program, such as an accredited practical nurse program or an institutional inservice training program for aides. Their orientation to their work setting and role is usually the responsibility of the professional nurse. Continuing education on a formal basis is also usually under the direction of the nurse, and the informal learning that takes place in the immediate work situation is largely the responsibility of the nurse also. Teaching and guiding instruction for allied nursing personnel, while time consuming, are vitally important aspects of the nurse's role and have a significant impact on the understanding and, ultimately, the quality of nursing care given. Not only is the nurse responsible for updating her own knowledge and skill in the area of nursing practice, but she is also responsible for sharing these updated skills with others who assist her.

If the nurse is employed in an agency that provides teaching and training programs, she will find that a considerable period of her time is spent in orienting and teaching others. The most common groups she will be involved with are student nurses, graduate nursing students, medical students, interns, residents, social work students, psychology interns, etc. In most settings, the nurse has no official or recognized responsibility for the education or training of these individuals. It is commonly acknowledged, however, that unofficially she has responsibility for this and will frequently be called upon to teach others about various aspects of the work environment and/or patient care.

The *condition of the patient* is the second variable in the scope of nursing practice. The nurse may provide care to individuals whose condition ranges from acutely ill to well. The needs of these patients influence the role the nurse plays in working with them [26]. For example, when the nurse cares for a seriously ill patient in the intensive care unit, she will provide the kind of supportive intervention that is necessary to improve his condition or to sustain life. This is quite different from her role in an ambulatory care setting, where patients are primarily healthy. In the acute care setting her role is one of caring for ill people who are receiving some form of treatment and/or are recuperating. In the ambulatory care setting her focus will be on maintaining patients in a healthy state and working toward prevention of illness. The first two variables in the conceptual model for nursing practice illustrate that the nurse has a diversity of roles which are guided by specific nursing behaviors.

The *environmental setting* is the third conditioning factor in the scope of nursing practice. "Just as any social organization develops its *mores* and *taboos,* so the social environment associated with the provision of health care strongly influences its conduct, and its results" [26]. Because the majority of nurses receive their initial education in the hospital setting, they tend to focus on the requirements needed to work with patients in these settings rather than in more disparate environments. For example, the nurse who works in a ghetto neighborhood clinic will be bound by very different guidelines than the nurse who works in an intensive care unit of a general hospital. The approach will depend on the differing needs of the patients, who may be located in unusual or unique surroundings and situations. The cultural and environmental differences can and do influence people in their acceptance or rejection of help [28]. The work environment, then, can be seen as a vital factor that contributes to the dynamic relationships between the other two variables in nursing practice, as illustrated in Figure 1.

Barriers to Effective Nursing Practice

It is clear that the practice of nursing is diversified and often complex. Diverse and complex factors create barriers that interfere with effective nursing practice. "Provision for full health service to the American public can be realized only when each health profession functions at its best" [29]. It is common knowledge that "nursing practice has long operated under unfavorable conditions" [30]. The position that nursing finds itself in today is not just a recent development. Specific patterns with accompanying problems impinge upon nursing practice and have dominated our profession for several generations; these patterns have been identified as: a nursing shortage, impoverished work environment and role misunderstanding [29].

Nursing Shortage: Real or Imagined?
For years now, we have heard about the nursing shortage throughout our country. Is it real or merely a misperception? The most recent statistics indicate that there are close to 1,200,000 registered nurses in the United States. Of that total number, almost 800,000, or 69 percent, are actively employed in nursing. Close to 400,000 nurses, or approximately 28 percent, are not employed [6]. These statistics immediately point out an inconsistency. Although the public, nursing leaders and others have constantly complained about the shortage of nurses, almost one out of every three registered nurses in this country is not working in her chosen profession.

When we ask whether or not the supply of nurses compares with the needs and demands projected by various experts and study groups, the outcome is rather surprising. The Lysaught report summarized various nursing manpower projections by a wide variety of groups. In almost every forecast of the number of nurses needed, the number of nurses being educated exceeded the projection slightly [31]. According to a survey of the number of budgeted vacant positions in nonfederal short-term general hospitals with at least 200 beds, the estimated vacancy rate of staff positions per hospital, for graduate nurses, declined from 8.8 percent in 1969 to 4.9 percent in 1971. This decline may imply either that there were more budgeted positions filled or fewer budgeted positions available [32]. If the majority of inactive nurses should decide to return to nursing, there would not be nearly enough positions available. Why, then, is there a prevailing viewpoint that a nursing shortage exists? As pointed out in the Lysaught report, the primary focus regarding the nursing shortage has been on the number of nurses who graduate every year. Because of these broad assumptions, policies and legislation have been enacted to increase the numbers of students entering nursing. Along with this, there has been an effort to increase the supply of allied nursing personnel. While expanding the numbers of nurses and nursing personnel may be a necessary goal, not enough attention has been directed to the continual high attrition rates in nursing, the question of need or demand and the distribution and utilization of personnel [33].

The most important question is, why *is* there such a high attrition rate in nursing, beginning with students who drop out of school to professional practitioners who become inactive? When one considers the preparation of nurses for the job market, it is a little like pouring sand in a hole that can never be filled up. We continue to educate more nurses to meet the increasing demands within the health care system. Yet, during the past decade, nurses have consistently dropped out.

"A profession is commonly distinguished by the fact that its members engage in active pursuit of their occupation during most of their lives" [34]. When compared to physicians, engineers, lawyers or teachers, nurses leave their profession at a much higher rate. With the exception of teaching, these other professions are composed mostly of males. As pointed out earlier, men value their work and others value men's work. Because most nurses are women, their work is not as valued. Also, our profession is subject to all the interruptions that are expected to take place among women: child-bearing and -rearing, household management and other marital responsibilities [34]. (The effect that the work environment has on attrition rates in nursing will be dealt with later.) Why is this, and does it really have to be this way? Do female nurses value their work? To answer these questions, we must backtrack.

To begin with, admission statistics for high school graduates in 1971–72 showed a higher percentage (6.2 percent) of females choosing nursing as a career. Over 6 percent of this total group chose nursing, the highest rate since the 1940s and 1950s [35]. Based on past experience, what can we predict will happen? The early socialization of these young women will become apparent and a significant number of graduates will probably drop out. As pointed out previously, a major goal promoted for American women is to achieve a rewarding and stable heterosexual relationship. Why, then, do so many women bother to choose nursing as a career? When a young person is asked what she wants to do when she grows up and she proudly replies, "I'm going to be a nurse," the response so often is something like, "Oh, that's nice, dear. That's a good thing for you to do until you find a husband [rich doctor]. And it'll make you a better wife and mother." This has been a prevailing attitude among nursing candidates as well. It is the usual pattern that many nurses marry young, have children and drop out of their profession. Many never find their way back. Character-istically, many women assign top priority to entering a successful heterosexual relationship that will lead to the development of the nuclear family along with all the old traditional responsibilities [36]. The nurse who drops out of the work world often lives as other women live, and she busies herself with child-rearing, house-keeping chores and possibly a hobby or two. It is not unusual to find these nurses volunteering their time for various projects such as blood drives, teaching first aid courses and the like. They rationalize that they are still involved in nursing. Some women who have dropped out of nursing have internalized a need to achieve and to be successful in other than the mother-wife role. Many say that they enjoy being a wife, that they love their husband and children, but that they feel empty and isolated much of the time. Once they resolve their guilt feelings, many of them return to the work world of nursing. For many women who make this decision, their lives are changed for the better; for others, it is a tragic mishap. An example will illustrate this.

Several years ago I was working in an intensive care unit, and a new staff nurse was hired to work part-time. I learned that she had graduated from a baccalaureate nursing program eight years previously but after graduation had married and worked less than a year as a staff nurse. When she quit work she had two children, both of whom were now in school. As her children were gone most of the day, they were not as dependent on her as they had been, and she was bored at home. She felt nervous and depressed a good bit of the time. With a great deal of anxiety, she enrolled in a two-week refresher course, which she successfully completed, and she was assigned to work in the intensive care unit, where she was to receive further orientation. On her third day at work, she was still petrified and unsure of herself in everything that she did. Although she received a great deal of support and encouragement from the other nurses, she was still very nervous and uncomfortable. At the end of the fourth day, she resigned and resolved she could never return. Her reason was that she had been out of nursing so long that it was a completely different world for her. And this was a woman in her late twenties who had excelled scholastically and clinically as a student. It would be easy to discount this incident as unusual, but is it? It might be said that the ICU is no place to resume working after having been away from nursing, but the entire health care system is changing continuously, and any area of nursing would require a great effort to "catch up." Two-week refresher courses help but will never make up for experience lost over a lengthy time span. The lost talent in this individual alone is considerable. She spent four years and a significant amount of money to prepare for a career in nursing, including an expensive college education. As almost half the students in colleges and universities today are women, until socialization patterns for both boys and girls change and until there are equal opportunities for women in the work world accompanied by shared child-rearing responsibilities, we will continue to see intelligent women wasting their talents.

Another factor that must be considered in relation to the high attrition rates in nursing is that of commitment. The goal for our profession should be to encourage women to view nursing as a lifelong career, just as other professions are viewed. Karen Lamb raises some fundamental issues regarding the commitment of many women who choose nursing as a career. First of all, she points out that we should concern ourselves with the *quality* of the woman who enters nursing. We must determine what nursing is for her. Does she want to contribute something to the profession? Is she willing to expend her time and talent, and if so, for how long? [37]. She states: "We must work to eradicate the notion that we are preparing other than the full professional" [38]. She strongly urges that an evaluation of the motivation and commitment of women be carried out prior to admitting them to schools of nursing. This is, admittedly, a difficult task. She suggests, however, that this might be accomplished through counseling sessions or some form of consciousness-raising. She further states: "If we are committed to the ideology of the egalitarian family over the traditional authoritarian, segmented family roles, then our practitioners must insist that husbands share the responsibility of the home" [39].

Lamb also points out that many of the nurses who drop out may do so from boredom, misguided vocational counseling, lack of challenge or frustration at not being able to become writers, researchers, doctors or lawyers. Again, it would be less costly to nursing in every respect to be more certain of the degree of com-

mitment and the quality of those who become nurses [40].
Lamb's appeal to members of our profession is that "We must
commit ourselves to educating practitioners for a life-time career,
not an interrupted, intermittent, half-hearted and uncommitted
practice of nursing" [41].

Since social changes of any significant magnitude are usually
slow in coming about, high attrition rates in nursing will probably
be with us for some time to come. The estimated average work
life of a nurse is between 20 and 21 years. When one considers
that a nurse can anticipate contributing to her profession for approximately 44 years, the tremendous waste of talent, energy
and experience within nursing becomes apparent. A work life
of 21 years represents only 48 percent of the total time available
[34]. This waste is unnecessary, but until women make a commitment to nursing as a lifelong career, until men share in child-
rearing and household tasks and until resocialization takes place,
health care and nursing practice will continue to be adversely
affected by a high "dropout" rate of nurses.

The improved technology and scientific advancements in health
science and the greater demand for services by consumers have
definitely increased the need for more quality nursing care. Future
studies carried out to project necessary nursing manpower must
focus on the trends, emphasis and needs related to health care.
Once this work has been evaluated, the appropriate distribution
and utilization of personnel can be determined. This has not yet
been done to any large degree.

Impoverished Work Environment
Earlier, it was pointed out that the work environment is an important variable affecting nursing practice. A major problem
identified in the Lysaught report was that the work environment
for nurses is *impoverished* [43]. "There is little doubt that low
salaries, poor working conditions, and lack of professional status
have led to the lack of commitment to nursing as a career and to
tangential problems in the numbers and distribution of personnel"
[44]. We need to look at these factors in greater depth in order
to understand their effects on nursing practice.

To begin with, for all but a small percentage of nurses, work
is carried out within a bureaucratic organization. Like other social

institutions, the health care system has experienced unprecedented growth in new knowledge and sophisticated technological advances. In order to use this information and skill to achieve the goals of large-scale, formal organizations such as health care institutions, bureaucratization has developed. "The type of organization designed to accomplish large-scale administrative tasks by systematically coordinating the work of many individuals is called a bureaucracy" [45]. Hospital and other health care institutions have developed into bureaucratic organizations over time. One of the reasons for this is the high degree of specialization that has developed in health care; this has created a need for a highly complex system of coordination [46]. Greater numbers of people are demanding health services, and a bureaucratic organizational structure is supposed to be more economical and efficient. The basic characteristics of a bureaucratic organization are as follows: "specialization; a hierarchy of authority; a system of rules; and impersonality" [47]. Bureaucracy "is a power instrument of the first order — for the one who controls the bureaucratic apparatus" [48].

While it would be impossible to deliver health services to the American public without some type of organized plan, the bureaucratic structure presents many problems that affect nursing practice. "The hierarchy of authority in a bureaucracy, essential for coordination, often produces among its lower echelons profound feelings of inequality and apathy that impede identification with the organization's objectives" [49]. These intense feelings of inequality have many effects detrimental to the operation of the organization. They lower interest in carrying out tasks and responsibilities to the person's maximum capabilities, inhibit identification with the organization and its objectives, destroy initiative and cut down the chances for solving emergent operating problems [50].

"Unless employees consider themselves partners in a common enterprise rather than tools in the hands of management, they are not prone willingly to assume responsibilities of their own" [50]. As previously pointed out, almost all institutions that employ nurses are dominated by a small group of administrators — the majority of whom are men. A bureaucracy characteristically concentrates power in the hands of a few individuals — usually men — and curtails the freedom of individuals that is so essential for democracy [51]. *Approximately 75 percent of all workers in health care are women* [52]. The majority of administrators are men. It would be impossible to provide health services to the American consumer without some form of bureaucratic organization to implement them. The problem with our present structure is that women, specifically nurses, are not considered partners of the men who are managing the health care institutions. They are merely led by them. Women's concerns and ideas are not considered to be as valid or important as those of their male health colleagues.

The findings of a recent survey conducted by Marjorie Godfrey for the journal *Nursing 75* support my previous comments. At random, 1,500 hospital-based nurses were selected from the *Nursing 75* subscription list; 500 were from Canada and the rest were from the United States. They were asked about the working conditions in their hospitals. In order to determine what aspects of the job were most dissatisfying to them, respondents were asked to rank all factors that bothered them. The results, with one exception, were fairly predictable. The most frequent complaint was inadequate staffing. Other complaints, ranked in descending order, were: low salaries, long or inconvenient working hours and shifts, poor physical working conditions, inadequate opportunities for advancement, small fringe benefits, and little job authority [53]. A surprising area of dissatisfaction that was overwhelmingly reported by nurses was an item not even included in the list of possible choices: "The biggest problem seems to be the bureaucracy, the hospital administration" [54]. Over and over in the survey, nurses reported a lack of communication with the hospital management. Nurses repeatedly wrote that the administration does not listen to of effectively deal with the various hospital problems. The large majority of nurses polled indicated that the management of their institutions pay little or no attention to them. When asked about communication between nurses and doctors, the medical staff fared slightly better than the administration. Only 21 percent stated communication was "great"; with physicians the majority (60 percent) answered "moderate"; 11 percent said "slight"; and 7 percent said it was "poor" [55].

Little attention is paid to the nurses' special concerns, and this has caused a great deal of dissatisfaction among them. As a result, a new wave of collective action and bargaining has been organized throughout the country to gain the attention of disinterested, unresponsive management.

Inadequate staffing was identified as one of the most dissatisfying aspects of the nurse's job; 75 percent of the respondents listed this as a major problem and 60 percent of the nurses believe there is a shortage of nurses in their area. Many commented that they had never worked anywhere that was not understaffed, which is doubtless true. Various studies and statistics along with budgeted positions indicate that the nursing shortage is not as great as it would seem (if we have one at all). Anyone who has recently worked in a hospital (general or psychiatric) or a nursing home will tell you very quickly, however, that the number of nurses available to provide direct patient care is inadequate. It is very frustrating to a nurse to leave her work day after day feeling guilty because she knows she should have done more for her patients. If only she could have had a few minutes more time to listen to them! Not listening to a patient may not be a matter of life or death for him, but it may affect his understanding of his illness or his psychological comfort.

The fact that a large percentage of the nurse's time is spent carrying out non-nursing tasks is one of the main reasons many nurses are dissatisfied with their working conditions. This is also a major impediment to effective nursing practice. In this same study, 84 percent of the nurses surveyed were expected to do non-nursing jobs such as stamping charts, cleaning equipment, answering telephones, relaying messages, etc. Most of the nurses indicated that they wanted to do what they were educated to do — give patient care [56]. The Lysaught report identified similar findings. Patients are deprived of 50 to 75 percent of the professional nurses' time in receiving care [57]. Patient care at times seems almost remote for the professional nurse, who is deluged with paperwork, administration, training and supervision for layers of assistants [44]. To counteract the perceived nursing shortage, many allied nursing personnel have been added to the health care system to extend the hands and skills of the professional nurse. In 1972, an estimated 427,000 licensed practical nurses [58] and 900,000 nurses' aides, orderlies and attendants were employed [27]. More and more of the nurses' time must be spent in training and supervising these individuals, leaving less and less time to spend in direct patient care. The nurse ends up giving care "through others." This is not fulfilling for the nurse because it interferes with the primary reason she chose nursing as a career. Inappropriate utilization of the skills and knowledge of the professional nurse is probably a frequent cause for nurses leaving nursing or for frequent changes in employment settings. It is a common complaint voiced by many nurses. Improper utilization of the professional nurse probably contributes most to the notion that there is a nursing shortage. Indeed, there is a shortage — but a shortage of professional nursing skill involved in direct patient care.

What about money matters? In the *Nursing 75* survey, nurses were asked if they felt their salary was adequate for the work they did. Surprisingly, 40 percent replied yes!; 59 percent replied no. Those who felt underpaid felt so because they have heavy responsibilities and work loads which are not adequately compensated. Many nurses feel that their salary is adequate when compared to that of other nurses but not so when compared to salaries in other professions or occupations because of the greater responsibility involved in nursing [59]. Since 1969, starting salaries for the "new graduate" employed in a staff nurse position has increased an average of 5.9 percent annually [60]. In 1972, the average starting salary for a staff nurse was $8,200 a year [61]. Since this represents an "average," one must keep in mind that even at this writing nurses in many sections of the country are still not earning salaries at this level. When one considers the annual rate of inflation over the past several years, it is obvious that salaries for nurses have not kept abreast with the rising cost of living. Last year, the inflation rate was 13 percent higher than the previous year. Very few nursing salaries went up proportionately. Two-thirds of the nurses who participated in the *Nursing 75* survey felt that $100 to $200 a month should be the increase over their present salaries. When the median salaries of various male-dominated occupations such as railroad conductors, real estate appraisers, auctioneers, electricians, plumbers and pipefitters, photographers, mail carriers, foresters, machinists (to name just a few) are compared with the median earnings of the female nurse, it is notable that the salaries of the former are all ranked higher than those of nurses [62]. While these male-intensive occupations are important and necessary, this comparison does point out the value our society places on services that are concerned with a traditionally feminine task (caring for others).

It was pointed out that "Joanne McCloskey, in her study of the influence of incentives on turnover rate, found that small salary raises would *not* have been effective in keeping nurses at jobs they left. Only when the raise amounted to $150 per month did it become significant enough to keep nurses on the job" [59]. This leads us to the next area of dissatisfaction identified by many nurses. Working schedules for most nurses are not comparable with the schedules of the majority of other workers in society. People who are ill require care 24 hours a day, seven days a week. This means that the majority of nurses do not have regularly scheduled days off, and they rotate over three different shifts. Only 3 percent of the nurses polled in the United States indicated that they had every weekend off. The majority of American nurses have every second or third weekend off, and 58 percent reported they are required to rotate shifts. Since the majority of nurses are married and have families, this type of sporadic work schedule contributes to their dissatisfaction with their work environment. Since we already know that child care is primarily the domain of women in our society, the working mother with a changing work schedule has special barriers to overcome. She must make arrangements for child care that allow for a very flexible and always changing schedule. The single nurse should not be overlooked either. It is difficult for her to arrange outside activities and her social life around a sporadic work schedule as well.

The overall results of the *Nursing 75* survey identified a basic philosophy among nurses. "Though most would welcome more autonomy, more attention and help from their management, as well as higher salaries, they want something else most, and many of them are willing to fight for it. That is the opportunity to give the best possible patient care" [63]. When nurses are not able to do this, they look for employment elsewhere. This leads to another chronic and major problem that plagues our profession and ultimately affects the practice of nursing — *turnover*.

On a national level, any gains that are made by employing new nurses or nurses who have been inactive are largely offset by losses that are experienced because of turnover. The national turnover ses is 70 percent. During a 12-month period, the health care facility has to replace seven out of every ten [64]. Some facilities have a 100 percent (or more) turnover rate. At the time the Lysaught report was completed, the estimated cost per replacement was $420 [64]. Today, it would be even greater. The cost in relation to the delivery of care and in terms of work organization is yet greater [64]. Why does this occur? It has been pointed out that this is an indication of "flight from an unhappy situation, followed by increasing frustration as the individual finds the next job — and the next — no different. It seems conceivable that many nurses find their assignments equally unsatisfying wherever they go" [64]. These factors combine to form what has been described as an impoverished work environment. Nurses seem to be always on the move in search of the ideal work setting where they can do what they were prepared to do — give patient care — in a way that they were ideally taught to do it. I predict that this pattern will continue until the work environment for nurses is enriched. Simply raising salaries will not remedy the problem. When the role of the nurse is better understood and respected, when the major responsibilities of nurses and of all women are more equally valued, when the basic issues and concerns of nurses are listened to, when nurses are given a voice in the decision-making process in the health care system, we will see the beginning of a true partnership with others develop. The result will be an improved work environment that will stimulate a long-term commitment by professional nurses.

This impoverished work environment is, of course, not the only reason for turnover. I recently conducted a survey within my own department to determine the main reasons nurses have left our institution. All employees were required to fill out a resignation form prior to their termination at the hospital, and the "reason" for terminating was requested along with other pertinent information. The data were compiled from these forms on all nurses who had resigned from January 1971 through June 1975. All the reasons given were listed and organized into 13 categories (Table 1). Since the hospital studied is fairly small, the total number of nurses terminating is relatively small. Still, while sweeping generalizations cannot be made from such a small population sample, the findings illustrate some interesting facts.

Table 1 Reasons Given by Professional Nurses for Terminating Their Employment at a Community Hospital from January 1971 — June 1975

Reason	Raw Number	Percentage	Rank
Job dissatisfaction	7	9.0	5
Better position	3	3.8	7
Better work hours/pay, etc.	2	2.6	8
Family responsibilities	8	10.3	4
Illness	2	2.6	8
Husband transferred job to new area	15	19.2	1
Continued education	9	11.5	3
Pregnancy	3	3.8	7
Moved to new area	13	16.7	2
Personal (no reason stated)	7	9.0	5*
Requested to terminate (poor performance)	6	7.7	6
Married and moved away	2	2.6	8
Miscellaneous	1	1.3	9
Total	N = 78	100.1	

*Includes only male nurse in study.

In the study, the most frequent reason that nurses gave for leaving was to relocate with their husbands. This is not a surprising finding, since it is common for families to move where the husband has the best job opportunity. It is difficult to find a married nurse who has relocated her husband and children because she had a better job opportunity in another area. Some enlightened couples are making career choices in specific areas on the basis of equal opportunities for both, however. Many of the married women who left our hospital to relocate because of their husband's job did so with regret. Two factors could explain why families relocate in accordance with job opportunities of the male. Men's work is more highly valued, and usually the male's earning potential is greater; therefore, it is economically more advantageous to consider the husband's job opportunities as a priority.

The second most frequently given reason for terminating was

The Indoctrination of Female Nurses

"moving to a new area." With the exception of one nurse, all the respondents in this category were single. Out of the singles group, three were widowed or divorced and had no family responsibilities. The other single nurses were all young. This group may be representative of many young people in America today. They are highly mobile and are searching for new experiences and adventure. The job market for nurses is virtually wide open throughout the country. Since these nurses have a skill that is in great demand, they are assured of a position in any number of locations and work settings. Since they have no family responsibilities, they are free to pursue their careers in many areas.

The next most frequently given reason for nurses terminating their employment was to continue their education. This corresponds with an increasing national trend in nursing to continue education on a formal basis [65]. Because the knowledge base in nursing is expanding and growing more complex, this trend should be encouraged and supported.

The fourth most frequent reason for termination was attributed to family responsibilities. This is not surprising because all these nurses were married and had children. Again, the responsibility for child-rearing and household management is considered the responsibility of women primarily. As long as this holds true, the nursing profession will continue to be affected by intermittent and/or inactive practitioners.

Job dissatisfaction and personal reasons were cited as causes for terminating employment by a significant number of nurses; the exact reasons were not always made clear. Because of this, one can only speculate on the specific causes. Perhaps, many nurses fear retribution if they are candid about their reasons for leaving. Certainly, this area should be investigated. We have attempted to do this at our facility by requesting an exit interview with each nurse who terminates her employment. It has been my experience that most nurses welcome this opportunity and are usually constructively critical about their employment experiences. They are equally candid about positive or rewarding experiences. Many nurses at our facility have pointed out problems similar to those highlighted in the *Nursing 75* study. While these nurses have been candid in talking about the many job dissatisfactions they experienced while employed at our center, in writing they frequently

give other reasons for terminating. Their oral comments support
the ideas expressed by many nurses in various studies and surveys,
and I am somewhat surprised that a greater percentage of nurses
do not list their specific reasons for leaving. Since "behavior speaks
louder than words," perhaps we have our greatest clues regarding
why nurses terminate their employment regardless of what they
put in writing.

A small percentage of nurses were requested to terminate their
employment on the basis of their work performance. In several
situations, the individuals had personal problems of such magnitude
that they were unable to carry out their responsibilities in a competent and safe manner.

Other reasons for leaving, cited by only a few nurses, were
better positions or pregnancy. In the first category, two of the
nurses who left for better positions ranked them as such because
they are now working the day shift with weekends off. Both have
family responsibilities, and such a schedule of course makes it
easier for them to manage both a career and a family. A third
nurse returned to a general hospital setting, which was her preferred area of practice.

Better work hours and/or pay, personal illness and marriage
were reasons given by a few nurses for terminating. Several
nurses included in the study returned at a later date and were re-
hired. Only one male nurse was included in the study. When
he terminated, he gave no reason; however, he did move to
another state.

This study involves only a small number of nurses in a rather
small agency located in a small city in middle America. It
would be unwise to generalize on the basis of an unsophisticated
survey. There are patterns here, however, that illustrate the
findings of other studies, and this type of information should
be used as a basis for changing those conditions in the work
environment that create frustration and dissatisfaction among
nurses.

I have focused on many factors in the work environment that
create barriers to nursing practice. So far, I have not focused on
the individual in the health care setting who has a major responsibility for the management of nursing practice — the director of
nursing. In most hospitals and nursing homes, the largest group of

The Indoctrination of Female Nurses

50 workers are the nursing staff. A director of nursing is usually responsible for organized nursing services. At first glance, it would seem that this individual holds a powerful position in the health care bureaucracy. Her department is usually the largest because it has the greatest number of people and provides a necessary service on a 24-hour basis. "In 1972, more than 1.3 million full and part-time registered nurses, licensed practical nurses, orderlies, aides and attendants worked in hospitals, most of them in the nursing services department. In public health agencies, a total of 82,546 full and part-time nursing service personnel were employed. In nursing and personal care homes, just over 400,000 full and part-time nursing service personnel were employed. In summary, about 2 million persons working full or part-time in 1972 were accountable for their work to one of the 26,952 nursing service administrators and assistants" [66]. Without the continuous service of the nursing director's department, hospitals, nursing homes and public health agencies would have to close down. From these facts, one might assume that a director of nursing has a powerful position, and within the almost all-woman organization, she does have power. Because most nursing departments are so large, there is usually a well-defined hierarchy within the department, and female nurses hold the majority of administrative positions throughout the hierarchy. It would therefore seem that nursing groups, and more specifically female nursing groups, have more autonomy than other groups [67].

As Virginia Cleland points out, however, "Nursing, in its utter isolation from all vestiges of power except within its own group, can be likened to the exploitation of Negroes in our culture. With women, as with Negroes, dominance is most complete when it is not even recognized" [67]. She makes an analogy between nursing today and the Southern black school principal in the separate educational system. He could advance within the all-black school system and become the "big man"; however, he would not have the same opportunity for upward mobility in an integrated system [68]. The director of nursing is in a similar position. She may have advanced through the nursing hierarchy by virtue of experience or advanced education to become the "big woman" in the all-woman system of nursing. That is as far as she will go, however, and her power in the health care system is limited to her own department. It must be understood that the top administrative positions in nursing are usually assigned with the approval of the male-dominated systems such as hospital administration and medicine [69]. The nurse administrator, of necessity, must report to the male authority systems all that is happening within the nursing community. She knows that much of what she can do within her department depends on the approval and support of the men who actually control the total system. Other nurses within the department see the director as a powerful person and therefore often choose her as a role model. They see the tremendous responsibilities she has, and they hear about the decisions she makes which they know affect them in their work situation. Some of them seek to emulate her in the future. What they do not see along with the responsibility is that the necessary authority is missing. For example, a director of nursing has the defined responsibility for managing the largest department in the health system with all the inherent problems that accompany so large a task. If one considers only two aspects of her responsibility — managing a 24-hour a day service and managing a large, diverse group of people to provide that service — it is easy to see the magnitude of her responsibility. Yet, the majority of directors of nursing do not manage or control their own departmental budgets. It is common knowledge that usually as much as half or more of the institution's total personnel budget is spent by the nursing department [70]. It is difficult to imagine many men who would accept such responsibility without the corresponding authority to go with it. Health care agencies are built and organized to provide a service to people. A director of nursing is hired to manage a department that will help provide the needed services. Then she is put in the position of so many housewives — she must ask permission to hire people and buy equipment that is needed to provide the service.

In our society, the individuals who control the pursestrings control others. They are the ones with the recognized power. This tells us once again where women — and nurses — stand: they are powerless. Many directors either do not recognize this, or are complacent about it or unable to do anything about it. Without radical and sweeping changes, this type of authority will remain limited to its own area and powerless in the larger health care system. "Unconsciously, in a search for autonomy and self-actualization, we

52 chose as our role models the Aunt Janes, who really have no power except over the hapless and are only female Uncle Toms" [69].

In light of the multiple problems pointed out by nurses with regard to their work environment, it is obvious that the management and communication skills of directors of nursing must be sophisticated and in tune with the problems of today. The American Nurses' Association has long recognized the critical issues and challenges that are facing the organized delivery of nursing services in this country. At a recent meeting, it was announced that "the profession identifies nursing administration as a vital force in designing and implementing a viable health delivery system. The leadership role of directors of organized nursing services is a critical one, if nursing is to achieve a substantive place in new and emerging health care systems" [71]. In order for the director better to fulfill her leadership role and to assume an equal share of the authority that will be needed to reshape the present health care system, she will have to expand her knowledge in several important areas. She must become knowledgeable in management and administrative methodology that deals with organizational systems and structures that effect change. She must learn to do long-range planning using new and innovative approaches to providing services. She must sharpen her communication skills to enable her to deal effectively with her colleagues, administrators and the public. She must acquire political sophistication in order to develop needed strategies for identifying nursing's contributions to organized health systems, the executive and legislative bodies and to the community at large. She must increase her knowledge regarding various relationships within the health care field. She needs an expanded awareness of consumer and community needs. This is a lot. We need not delude ourselves into thinking that it will be easy to bring about the changes that are so desperately needed. If the nurses in leadership roles will accept the challenges and commit themselves to the risks involved in facing the issues, they will serve as strong role models for younger nurses just entering our profession. Women everywhere have suffered from the lack of achievement-oriented female models who have attained successful leadership roles. Those women already established in leadership positions have a special responsibility now in this period when the traditional role of women is being challenged and defined. They not only must prove that they are intelligent and have leadership ability, but they must also help other women to develop their self-confidence and their talents. Remaining oblivious to their lack of power will do nothing to improve their lot.

Throughout this book, it is pointed out that sex discrimination is a pervasive problem for women nurses and for the entire female population. It permeates everywhere and it affects our profession. Many of the factors that have been emphasized have been the results of outside forces or groups. That in itself is irritating and difficult to deal with. It is perhaps even more annoying to have to admit that we promote discrimination on the basis of sex *within* our profession. According to data compiled in 1972, male nurses are *twice* as apt to become administrators or assistants as women [72]. Less than 2 percent of all nurses are men, and yet of the 11,000 actively employed, just under 8 percent of them are administrators or assistants; only 4 percent of the women nurses employed are administrators or assistants [72]. Not only do men in nursing have an edge over women in filling administrative leadership positions, but they fare better economically when all nurses' salaries are compared. According to the Bureau of Labor Statistics of the United States Department of Labor, the median annual earnings for male registered nurses in 1969 was $7,013. For women registered nurses, it was $5,603 annually [73]. Although I have emphatically stated that work carried out by women, such as nursing, is not as valued as work carried out by men, these statistics indicate that when men carry out nursing tasks, the tasks are more highly valued and the remuneration is greater. Apparently, blatant sexism and inequality in the work situation are just as prevalent in our female-dominated profession as in every other profession or occupation.

Our profession should encourage many more men to choose nursing as a career. Caring for people gives one a sense of fulfillment and would certainly enrich the lives of many men in our society if they were free to choose nursing as a way of providing service to others. Both men and women are in need of care, and both men and women have the capacity to give that care. To reward men to a greater degree for giving that care simply because they happen to be men is ludicrous as well as demoralizing to

at this occurs in our profession comes as no
terns for this seem to be formed early in our
the professional student nurse organization on the
national level, a significant number of the elected
board members are male students. These men surely
blamed for this outcome because the overwhelming
majori, of the members who vote them into office are women.
This supports the theory that women as well as men are socialized
to believe that men are natural leaders, and it is a philosophy reinforced throughout the entire nursing community. Women who
are an obvious minority in male-dominated professions do not
have the same advantages as men in nursing. In fact, the opposite
holds true except on rare occasions.

I have talked with male nurses who do not enjoy these special
privileges. Several have told me that they have often felt "used,"
meaning that they feel more is expected of them by their women
colleagues in regard to leadership roles simply because they are
men. Often they feel that this puts special pressures and expectations on them that they do not desire. Some women have gone so
far as to suggest that the way for nursing to become appropriately
recognized and legitimatized is to recruit more men; then we will
gain proper recognition and status. This would not only be unfair
to the men in nursing but it would be the greatest "cop-out" in
history for American nurses. It would merely perpetuate the
dominant stereotype about women as the weaker, powerless sex.
Yes, we need more men in nursing, but they should receive no
more or no less than their women colleagues.

Role Misunderstanding
Another major problem that creates a barrier to effective nursing
practice is that of role misunderstanding of the professional nurse.
The nurse's role, it seems, is misunderstood by just about everyone.
To the lay public, to hospital administrators and to many physicians
and other health care workers, a nurse, is a nurse, is a nurse. In a
general hospital, often anyone in white is considered to be "a
nurse." In other settings, such as psychiatric facilities and public
health agencies, where uniforms may or may not be worn, the
perception of the nurse is still a stereotype — she gives pills or
takes temperatures. This role confusion stems from several factors.

To begin with, other than nurses themselves, many people do 55not realize that there are three different types of educational programs that prepare professional nurses. Moreover, nursing is the only profession in which the members are prepared in three different ways and the end-product is called by the same name — a registered nurse. A graduate nurse may have completed (1) a diploma program in a hospital school, (2) an associate degree program in a junior college or (3) a baccalaureate program in a college or university. However, in most work settings, all nurses do similar work. The public is confused about this. Hospital administrators, directors of nursing, physicians and others seem to be equally confused because they continue to expect all three types of nurses to function similarly. In the meantime, nursing educators, along with many other nurses, are still heatedly arguing over which one of these types of nurse is the "best."

While the philosophies of each of these educational programs purport to prepare a different *level* of functioning practitioner, the graduates enter the real work world and are all assigned basically similar tasks. The agencies that employ these various practitioners have not updated their standards of practice and role expectations in accordance with the educational preparation of the nurse. The graduate nurse knows what she has been prepared to do. When she sees the confusion of those around her and within the system, she becomes confused also. It is probably safe to say that this role misunderstanding has its roots in our own professional education system.

As I have already pointed out, nursing is a dynamic profession that is ever changing in an attempt to meet dynamic and increasing health care needs. Because of this, great diversification in the nursing role is emerging. Some of these aspects have already been discussed. We are now seeing a greater development of clinical specialization, as well as significant alterations in reciprocal roles of nurses and other health care workers, particularly physicians [74]. It has been pointed out that nurses could provide one of the solutions to "the known shortcomings of a health system in which one out of four persons is receiving less than adequate care" [75]. More highly specialized, expanded roles for nurses could contribute, and in many instances have, to the upgrading of care for large sections of the growing population [75]. A major emphasis in nursing has been health-teaching, in an effort to maintain good health and as a preventive measure. These new roles are not well understood or are not well publicized and therefore add to the confusion as to what the role of nursing really is or should be.

While new and expanded roles are developing for nurses, general confusion remains about the usual role of the nurse, who is viewed as either having very specific, technical tasks or very global, all-encompassing responsibilities. This perception of the nurse is perpetuated because her skills are often inappropriately utilized in the work situation, and she ends up doing a little bit of everything. Television, magazines and books do little toward correcting the misperceived and misunderstood role of the nurse. Nurses themselves are guilty of making their roles confusing to others. They do not often enough take the initiative to teach others, particularly patients and co-workers, about the varied and important aspects of their work.

Probably one of the most significant factors contributing to role misunderstanding in nursing is the conspicuous general lack of knowledge regarding the importance of good nursing practice. The efforts of a nurse are less conspicuous than the dramatic results of surgery and are more apt to be overlooked [76]. "Everyone 'knows' that nurses are vital to health processes, but the general and occupational views of nursing scarcely look on nursing care as crucial to the outcome of treatment" [76]. Significant findings have been documented to indicate that "quality nursing care can (a) improve the actual treatment accorded the patient; (b) improve the economics connected with the delivery of health care; and (c) provide the personal reinforcement needed by the nurses themselves to deepen their commitment to the field" [76]. The fact that many people, including nurses themselves, do not recognize the potential or actual contributions of quality nursing practice has helped to perpetuate the misunderstandings surrounding the role of the nurse. What is needed is more research to document the effects of good nursing practice, followed by wide dissemination of this information. Only when nurses themselves, the general public and other health care workers know, understand and appreciate the meaningful contributions of nurses will the practice of nursing be more highly valued.

1. Lamb, Karen T. Freedom for Our Sister, Freedom for Ourselves: Nursing Confronts Social Change. *Nursing Forum,* Vol. 12, No. 4, 1973, p. 328.
2. Worthington, Nancy L. National Health Expenditures, 1929–74. *Social Security Bulletin,* February 1975, p. 3.
3. Lysaught, Jerome P. *An Abstract for Action, National Commission for the Study of Nursing and Nursing Education.* New York: McGraw-Hill, 1970, p. 8.
4. Ibid., p. 11.
5. Ibid., p. 26.
6. American Nurses' Association. *Facts About Nursing 72–73.* Kansas City, Mo.: American Nurses' Association, 1974, p. 6.
7. Ibid., p. 7.
8. Sommers, Dixie. Occupational Rankings for Men and Women by Earnings. *Monthly Labor Review,* United States Department of Labor, Bureau of Labor Statistics, August 1974, p. 2.
9. Lysaught, op. cit., p. 110.
10. Group, Thetis M., and Roberts, Joan I. Exorcising the Ghosts of the Crimea. *Nursing Outlook,* Vol. 22, No. 6, June 1974, p. 369.
11. Ibid., p. 368.
12. Ibid., p. 371.
13. Cleland, Virginia. Sex Discrimination: Nursing's Most Pervasive Problem. *American Journal of Nursing,* Vol. 71, No. 8, August 1971, p. 1547.
14. Group, op. cit., p. 373.
15. Ibid., p. 372.
16. Lysaught, p. 58.
17. Lambertson, Eleanor. The Changing Role of Nursing and Its Regulation. *Nursing Clinics of North America,* Vol. 9, No. 3, September 1974, p. 396.
18. Ibid., p. 397.
19. Ibid., p. 399.
20. Heide, Wilma Scott. Nursing and Women's Liberation — A Parallel. *American Journal of Nursing,* Vol. 73, No. 5, May 1973, p. 824.
21. Group, op. cit., p. 370.
22. Lysaught, op. cit., p. 121.
23. Ibid., pp. 64–65.
24. Ibid., p. 65.
25. Ibid., p. 66.
26. Ibid., p. 67.
27. American Nurses' Association, op. cit., p. 181.
28. Lysaught, op. cit., pp. 67–68.
29. Ibid., p. 49.
30. Ibid., p. 75.
31. Ibid., pp. 50–51.
32. American Nurses' Association, op. cit., p. 22.
33. Lysaught, op. cit., p. 53.

58   34. Ibid., p. 33.

35. American Nurses' Association, op. cit., p. 70.

36. Bardwick, Judith M., and Douvan, Elizabeth. Ambivalence — the Socialization of Women. In *Woman in Sexist Society: Studies in Power and Powerlessness,* Gornick, Vivian, and Moran, Barbara (Eds.). New York: Basic Books, 1971, p. 235.

37. Lamb, op. cit., p. 339.

38. Ibid., p. 340.

39. Ibid., p. 341.

40. Ibid., p. 344.

41. Ibid., p. 342.

42. Cleland, op. cit., p. 1542.

43. Lysaught, op. cit., p. 55.

44. Ibid., p. 56.

45. Blau, Peter M. *Bureaucracy in Modern Society.* New York: Random House, 1968, p. 14.

46. Ibid., p. 17.

47. Ibid., p. 19.

48. Ibid., p. 21.

49. Ibid., p. 69.

50. Ibid., p. 80.

51. Ibid., p. 114.

52. Waldman, Elizabeth, and McEaddy, Beverly J. Where Women Work: An Analysis by Industry and Occupation. *Monthly Labor Review,* U.S. Department of Labor, Bureau of Labor Statistics, May 1974, p. 3.

53. Godfrey, Marjorie. Working Conditions: How Do Yours Compare with Other Nurses? *Nursing 75,* Vol. 5, No. 5, May 1975, p. 90.

54. Ibid., p. 91.

55. Ibid., p. 92.

56. Ibid., p. 98.

57. Lysaught, op. cit., p. 57.

58. American Nurses' Association, op. cit., p. 166.

59. Godfrey, op. cit., p. 100.

60. American Nurses' Association, op. cit., p. 130.

61. Ibid., p. 131.

62. Sommers, op. cit., pp. 37–39.

63. Godfrey, op. cit., p. 102.

64. Lysaught, op. cit., p. 133.

65. American Nurses' Association, op. cit., p. 108.

66. Arnold, Pam. Nurse Administrators Profiled: Big Job, Low Pay. *American Nurse,* Vol. 7, No. 4, April 1975, pp. 2, 7.

67. Cleland, op. cit., p. 1543.

68. Ibid., pp. 1543–1544.

69. Ibid., p. 1544.

70. Ibid., p. 1545.

71. Flaherty, Agnes. Group Is Key in Delivery of Health Care. *American Nurse,* Vol. 7, No. 4, April 1975, p. 1.
72. Ibid., p. 2.
73. Sommers, op. cit., pp. 39, 43.
74. Lysaught, op. cit., p. 69.
75. Ibid., p. 70.
76. Ibid., p. 73.

3   How Do I Love Me?

Carol Spengler

*We should not pity the strong.
We should love them, for they
have a terrible need of love [1].*

Victoria Ocampo

These words by Victoria Ocampo at first sound dichotomous, but this quote has a special meaning because it is especially pertinent to women. Although women in our society have been socialized into rigid roles, they are very strong. The fact that society has not yet recognized the strength, the character and the potential of women does not prove that women lack these characteristics, and they need love as do all human beings. Women in fact have *special* needs for love that will be explored in this chapter. Many of these special needs are based on how women perceive themselves. How we love ourselves has as much to do with our perception of ourselves as any other factor. How we perceive ourselves can largely be attributed to our early life experiences and our socialization process. How much and in what ways we love ourselves have a great bearing on our behavior and ultimately whether or not we see ourselves as strong. This chapter, then, is about love. How we love ourselves as women and as nurses affects all that we do. It is important to explore the question "How do I love me?" in order to understand ourselves better. The answer

62 to this question also provides us with clues as to why nurses and women in the other walks of life occupy their present-day positions in our society.

The emotion called love has perplexed people down through the ages, but very few empirical studies of love have been conducted. More studies are needed on the concept of love, to enlighten us and to increase our understanding of it. Hopefully, the results of these studies would be our learning to love more deeply, completely and maturely. Because love is a complex concept, it is not easy to answer the question "What is love?" We know that we experience many different kinds of love. Many of our loves coexist and nourish one another as well as conflict with one another at times. "The future of any one love depends upon its place in the complex pattern of all our loves" [2]. When we speak of love in a general way, it can be defined as the ability to form satisfying and meaningful relationships with other human beings [2]. In a broader sense, it may be defined as any kind of attachment which may be to a person, a place, an idea, an object, an activity or even to oneself [2]. Love is an active power in people; a power that both breaks through the walls which separate individuals from others and unites them with others. Love makes people overcome their sense of isolation and separateness, and it also permits them to be themselves and to retain their integrity [3]. Erich Fromm has described the active character of love as primarily *giving,* not receiving. He points out, however, that there is widespread misunderstanding concerning this "giving." Many people interpret giving as "giving up" something, sacrificing or being deprived of something. For some, the notion that it is better to give than to receive means that there is more virtue in suffering deprivation than in experiencing joy. For others, giving is interpreted differently. To them, giving is the highest expression of potency. "In the very act of giving, I experience my strength, my wealth, my power. This experience of heightened vitality and potency fills me with joy. I experience myself as overflowing, spending, alive, hence as joyous. Giving is more joyous than receiving, not because it is a deprivation, but because in the act of giving lies the expression of my aliveness" [3]. In the act of giving, something is born, and the individuals involved are grateful for the life that is born for each of them. With regard to love, this then means that love is a power which produces love. On the other hand, impotence is the inability to produce love [3].

Erich Fromm also identified basic elements that are common to all forms of love. These are *care, responsibility, respect* and *knowledge*. Love in relation to the first element, *care,* is shown by the active concern for the life and growth of that which we love. Concern and care then imply another aspect of love and that is *responsibility.* In this sense, responsibility is the response to needs, expressed or unexpressed, of another human being. It is entirely a voluntary act as opposed to a duty imposed from outside forces. Fromm points out that responsibility could easily turn into possessiveness and domination if it were not for the third aspect of love, which is *respect.* Respect is the ability to see individuals as they are and to be aware of their individual uniqueness. Respect does not mean fear and awe, and it implies the absence of exploitation. When we love others, we feel one with them as they are, not as we need them to be. It is only possible for us to respect others when we ourselves have achieved independence. Only on the basis of freedom is respect able to exist. It is not possible to respect a person unless we first know him or her. We gain *knowledge* of others when we transcend the concern we have for ourselves and see others in their own terms [3].

All these aspects of love — care, responsibility, respect and knowledge — are mutually interdependent and are found in the mature person who productively develops his own power, who has given up narcissistic dreams of omnipotence, who wants only what he has actually worked for and who has acquired humility based on inner strength [3]. The ability to love is viewed then as one of the important characteristics of a well-adjusted individual.

Our ability to love is not something that is fixed and finite when we are born. We must learn to love. Many of our life experiences, especially those in early life, affect our ability to love. All of us as children went through the same stages of development. Our different experiences as we went through these stages, however, had an individual effect on our overall development and ultimately on our ability to love. These experiences also affected our capacity as adults to give and receive love. No two individuals reach adulthood with the same capacities to love and to be loved. This is one reason it is difficult to study the emotion love. These individual differences also contribute to confusion in understanding people who are significant to us, such as parents, children and other relatives, co-workers, friends, etc. Our success in many differing relationships depends to a large degree on our understanding and recognizing individual differences in the capacity to love. Also, our previous loves influence any particular love that we may have today. Whether our past experiences with various types of love were positive or negative determines how we will approach a new opportunity for love. "The way we relate ourselves each day to people, places, and events is an integral part of our life. Our ability to love is expressed in and is affected by *all* our relationships; not merely the rare, romantic one we isolate as good enough to call love" [2].

There are so many kinds of love: parental love, romantic love, brotherly and sisterly love, friendship love, etc. The basic and most essential love, however, is self-love. All too often self-love is associated with unpleasant ideas. Many times we confuse self-love with selfishness and other negative connotations. The fact is that all other subsequent loves suffer if we do not accept and enjoy our primary attachment — the love of the self. When our emotional growth is impaired and unhappy, we become enslaved by the demands of the self, which results in our failing to enjoy being with others or being alone. A necessary condition for the enjoyment of the love of others is a positive attitude toward the self [2]. "We build all our other loves on the love we have for ourselves, and the quality of all our other loves depends upon the quality of this initial love" [2]. Learning to love begins at birth. The first kind of love that we develop is our self-love. The infant's first attachment is to himself. At first the young infant is unable to distinguish the boundaries of his own person. Over time, the infant begins to discover his own identity, which is separate from others. "We begin to think well or poorly of ourselves at the same time that we learn to recognize the very existence of ourselves. Our initial attachment to ourselves begins tinged with positive or negative feelings" [2].

Self-esteem, then, is the "evaluation which the individual makes and customarily maintains with regard to himself: it expresses an attitude of approval or disapproval, and indicates the extent to which the individual believes himself to be capable, significant, successful and worthy. In short, self-esteem is a personal judgement of worthiness that is expressed in the attitudes the individual holds toward himself" [4]. The individual conveys this subjective experience to others through overt expressive behavior and by verbal descriptions. The attitudes that the individual holds toward himself may be conscious or unconscious like other orientations and dispositions. The attitude the individual holds toward himself will be expressed in his posture, voice, gestures and performance [4].

The *self* is one's inner world which is the result of evaluational interaction with others. We know that the self-concept is shaped and formed to a large degree in the earlier period of childhood. It is developed through interaction with people and the individual's total environment. As the self-concept develops, it permits the individual to act, to adjust, to make decisions and to personalize his reactions [5]. The self "is a composite of a person's thoughts and feelings, strivings and hopes, fears and fantasies, his views of what he is, what he has been, what he might become, and his attitudes pertaining to his worth" [5]. Quite simply, our self-concept is how we perceive ourselves.

Those individuals who have had a greater focusing on negative feelings will develop an "undervalued" self. There are many examples of human behavior that illustrate the development of a poor or undervalued self-concept. Such behavior falls into two main categories. The inability to live up to one's potential, or "under-performance," is the first category. "The person who thinks poorly of himself shrinks his aspirations to a level below his ability and even his ability is frequently impaired by the distraction and discouragement of his intense self-concern" [2].

The second category is labeled a sense of unworthiness. This is not the same as humility or modesty. It is self-depreciation. Individuals who do not like themselves are apt to retreat in advance from their own fear of rejection. As a result, their potential is never fully met. "The self we live with is our own, and how we live with others is no better or worse than how we live with that self" [2]. The attitude we have toward ourselves colors our relationships with others, and the more important the relationships are, the more marked the coloration.

Since we know that negative response and feedback contribute to poor self-esteem, what specifically should be done to foster positive self-love? To begin with, the child needs an abundance of praise and approval from those who are significant in his world. The opportunity for self-expression and creativity must be fostered. Attention and praise when the child successfully achieves some task reinforces a sense of positive self-love. In a climate that is more encouraging than critical, more approving than disapproving, the child has a greater opportunity for discovering himself and seeing himself in a positive way. All of us had to learn as children that there were limits to our abilities in many directions. We also discovered that we had specific skills in different areas. How good we felt about ourselves affected how we adjusted to our personal strengths and weaknesses. Those who have developed a strong sense of self-love approach life with a feeling of adequacy. These individuals do not spend a great amount of time focusing on themselves. They love themselves, are comfortable with themselves and enjoy being involved with others. That is not to imply that life is easy for these people. Individuals who have a healthy love for themselves are able to cope with the ordinary pressures, conflicts and stresses in life more effectively. Because they believe in themselves and have a feeling of adequacy, they are able to approach life and its problems in general with a sense of self-confidence. When things do not go well, they are able to cope and to adjust to the situation. Also present in these individuals is a self-acceptance. They accept themselves for who they are and what they are. This does not mean that they passively accept all that is happening around them or within themselves. They have realistic and specific dissatisfactions with themselves and their environment. Instead of merely complaining, however, they seek new knowledge, skills, understanding and insights in order to change that which they are dissatisfied with. Because these individuals like themselves, they are more apt to judge themselves kindly. The more kindly they are in judging themselves, the more kindly they are in judging

others [2]. In short, the individual who loves himself is better
able to love others. This love for self and others enhances one's
ability to be constructively critical and therefore to solve problems
effectively. Self-love, then, rather than limiting and enslaving the
individual, actually liberates him [2].

Long ago, Maslow identified what he considered to be basic
motivational needs for all human beings. These basic needs are
for: life, safety, security, belongingness and affection, respect
and self-respect and self-actualization [6]. The highest level of
achievement in regard to our basic needs is eventually to progress
in our development until we become a self-actualized individual.
This is considered to be the epitome of a healthy, mature adult.
Individuals who eventually become self-actualized are said to have
adequately satisfied their other basic needs for safety, belongingness,
love, respect and self-esteem. As pointed out earlier, our self-love
affects all that we do and all that we become; therefore, the degree
to which we achieve these needs is dependent on our self-love.

Becoming a self-actualized person is a goal that is valued in our
society, and yet many people feel that it is a difficult one to attain.
Since it is a dynamic rather than static process, self-actualization
changes throughout life. The process involved in becoming self-
actualized goes on all the time in the life history of the individual.
When this fact is known, then, it becomes clear that it is not really
a matter of *being* a self-actualized person but rather that we are
always *becoming* self-actualized [6].

What does it mean to become a self-actualized person and why is
it considered important? Self-actualization, according to Maslow,
is an ongoing actualization of potentials, talents and capacities. It
is the fulfillment of one's mission. It is a fuller knowledge of and
acceptance of the individual's own intrinsic nature. It is also an
unceasing trend toward unity, synergy or integration within the
individual [6]. He further defines self-actualization as "an episode,
or a spurt in which the powers of the person come together in a
particularly efficient and intensely enjoyable way, and in which he
is more integrated and less split, more open for experience, more
idiosyncratic, more perfectly expressive or spontaneous, or fully
functioning, more creative, more humorous, more ego-transcending,
more independent of his lower needs, etc. He becomes in these
episodes more truly himself, more perfectly actualizing his

68 potentialities, closer to the core of his Being, more fully human" [7]. Rather than being an all-or-none affair, this definition points out that self-actualization is a matter of degree and frequency. We should not assume that only the most extraordinary person becomes self-actualized, for probably in most life histories episodes of self-actualization have occurred [6]. It is easy to see why becoming a self-actualized person is an important goal. Moving toward self-actualization means achieving our highest level of our motivational development in regard to our most basic human needs. It is also important to recognize that all of us, given the opportunity and appropriate support, have the potential for becoming self-actualized individuals.

Along with becoming a self-actualized person, it is also widely recognized that a healthy, mature adult should strive toward developing autonomy. Being autonomous means that the individual is self-governing. He also discards patterns that are inappropriate and irrelevant to living in the present [8]. Almost everyone has the capacity to become autonomous. Again, as with the process of self-actualization, developing autonomy is an ongoing process. According to James and Jongeward, three important capacities that have been demonstrated in those who are autonomous are: awareness, spontaneity and intimacy [8]. The autonomous person is aware of what is happening around him. His perception of the world around him is based on his own personal experiences rather than the way someone taught him to perceive it. He also knows his inner world of fantasies and feelings and yet, he is not ashamed or afraid of them. Because he is aware, he also hears other people. In summary, he knows where he is, what he is doing and how he feels about it [8].

The autonomous person has the capacity to be spontaneous. In his spontaneity, he has the freedom to see the many options that are open to him and to choose the ones that are appropriate to his particular situation and his goals. He is liberated and does not compulsively live a predetermined life-style. His choices give purposeful direction to his own potentialities. Because he consciously decides for himself what he will do, he is *free*.

Another important capacity seen in the autonomous person is that of intimacy. Intimacy is expressing warmth, tenderness and closeness to others. In the process of sharing thoughts and feelings at a deeper level, the individual becomes more open and is able to reveal more of his real self. He also recognizes the uniqueness in others and does not try to change this as he relates closely to the individual. In summary, the autonomous individual is primarily concerned with "being." He is concerned with *being more* rather than getting more [8].

So far, I have attempted to define and illustrate general concepts concerning the complex emotion called love. I have pointed out that the ability to develop many varied loves throughout our lifetime is influenced by our most basic and essential love which is self-love. The individual who develops a healthy love for himself will approach life with a sense of worthiness and self-confidence. This is important, as it enhances the individual's potential for becoming an autonomous, self-actualized individual. Becoming autonomous and self-actualized is recognized as being the ultimate level of development for the healthy, mature adult. In short, it means that the individual maximizes and achieves his own innate potential to become the kind of individual he wants to be. He therefore takes responsibility for himself. He also relates effectively to others who are significant in his life experiences. In a general sense, it could be said that this individual has the potential for becoming a "winner" in life.

As we look around us every day, we can identify many individuals who are winners. Unfortunately, we also see individuals who could be termed *losers*. The slang terms *winners* and *losers* have many different connotations in our culture. The traditional definition of "beating or being beaten by others" is not the meaning that I am referring to. Instead, I prefer the definitions of James and Jongeward. They have defined a winner as "one who responds authentically by being credible, trustworthy, responsive and genuine, both as an individual and as a member of a society" [8]. Losers are those individuals who fail to respond authentically [8]. Focusing on characteristic behaviors of individuals who could be described as winners or losers is relevant because it enhances our awareness and, hopefully, our understanding of human behavior as it relates to love. Ultimately, our capacity to love, including our ability to love ourselves, affects how we function as human beings. Later in the chapter, I hope to illustrate how all these ideas relate specifically to nurses as well as women in the world as a whole.

70   No individual is totally a winner or totally a loser. Winners and losers, however, do have characteristics that have been identified by James and Jongeward. Let us focus on people who could be labeled winners. To a winner, achievement is not the most important thing in the world. The most important thing is authenticity. Because winners are authentic people, they experience the reality of themselves by knowing themselves well and feeling comfortable in being themselves. They actualize their own uniqueness and at the same time appreciate the uniqueness of others. Winners live their lives as "themselves" rather than as they feel they "should be." Winners reveal their real selves instead of projecting images that are expected or desired by others. They know the difference between being loving and acting loving, being stupid and acting stupid, being knowledgeable and acting knowledgeable. Winners are not afraid of being autonomous — they enjoy it and thrive on it. They have faith in themselves even though they may fail at times. Winners enjoy using their own knowledge and their own thinking. They admire and respect others but are not totally awed, defined, demolished or bound by others. They don't pretend to be helpless. They take responsibility for their own life because they are their own boss and they know it. They have a sense of timing and therefore respond appropriately to different situations. Time is precious to winners and therefore they do not kill time. They live in the present; however, they are aware of experiences from the past and look forward to the future. Winners are aware of their own feelings and limitations but are not afraid of them. They are able to love and to be loved by others. Winners are enjoyable to be around because they are able to be spontaneous; they do not have to respond to situations in rigid, predetermined ways. They have a zest for life. Winners not only enjoy their own accomplishments but they enjoy the accomplishments of others. Winners enjoy themselves but are also able to discipline themselves when necessary. They do not get their security by controlling others. They do not set themselves up to lose. Winners care about the world and its people. They are compassionate, concerned individuals who are committed to improving the quality of life. In the face of adversity, winners do not see themselves as totally powerless. They will do what they can to make the world around them a better place [8].

In contrast, losers are individuals who do not succeed in making the transition from total helplessness as infants to independence and interdependence as adults. They avoid becoming self-responsible. They hang on to manipulative techniques that they learned early in life to cope with negative experiences. Losers are a bore — even to themselves. They seldom live in the present because they are busily occupied with the past or the future. They feel sorry for themselves and blame others and excuse themselves for their unsatisfactory experiences in life. Their ability to deal effectively with the real world is hampered because their perceptions of what is going on are incorrect or incomplete. Losers spend a great deal of time play-acting. They pretend, manipulate and perpetuate old roles from childhood. They repress the capacity to express spontaneous ranges of possible behavior. Because they are afraid to try new things, they maintain their own status quo. They are repeaters — they repeat their own mistakes and those of their culture. Losers have difficulty giving and receiving affection. Honest, intimate relationships with others are difficult, if not impossible. Losers do not use their intellect appropriately and as a result much of their potential lies dormant. They rationalize and intellectualize about their actions [8]. Unless they recognize their loser characteristics and work toward becoming winners, these individuals have little hope of becoming autonomous, self-actualized individuals. Life for them will be disappointing and sour.

Historically, as our society has become more civilized, philosophers, theologians, scientists, poets and others have attempted to define the meaning and purpose of our existence. Many theories have been developed to explain our evolutionary process as human beings. As our knowledge increases about the mysterious aspects of our humanness, older theories are replaced with new ideas. More and more people are concerned with understanding not only the biophysiological aspects of human beings but all aspects of human behavior. In many ways, it is much easier to analyze and synthesize the physical aspects of human beings than the behavioral aspects. In spite of this, a great deal has been written and hypothesized about human behavior and its development. As pointed out, the concept of love as it relates to human beings is complex. The various theories identified in this chapter pertain to all human beings. No differentiation is made on the basis of sexual differences.

72   When we talk about our capacities to love and those things which influence our capacity to love, it is assumed that these ideas hold true for all human beings regardless of their sex. The basic needs identified in relation to love are human needs — not masculine or feminine needs. As women, we have learned that when scholars refer to "mankind" and they use the pronoun "he," members of both sexes are meant. Likewise, when we ourselves write we too refer to both sexes, out of habit and for the sake of brevity, in masculine terms. We have learned to integrate "he" to mean "me too." Or have we?

If Maslow's theory regarding basic human needs is indeed true and the highest level of achievement for the healthy, mature person is to become a self-actualized adult, how do women as a group fare? Are the majority of women functioning as autonomous, self-actualized adults? Are the majority of men functioning this way? The answer is that some women do function as autonomous, self-actualized individuals. Unfortunately, when one considers the role, the position and the functions of the majority of women in our society, it is quite apparent that most women do not have the same opportunity as men to develop into this type of individual. No, the vast number of American women are not autonomous. In contrast, a great number of men do function autonomously and certainly have a much greater opportunity to become self-actualized individuals. Recall that our ability to love and be loved begins with learning to love ourselves. This self-love will affect all that we do and become. It will certainly affect our ability to become an autonomous, self-actualized individual. Should we accept the notion that women are simply different from men and therefore inferior? Is anatomy destiny? Definitely not. The answer can again be found in the way in which women are defined in society and ultimately the way we feel about ourselves.

Alterity of Women in Society

Simone de Beauvoir pointed out that women have been established as "the other" in society. This concept of *alterity* or *otherness* of women is illustrated in many ways. To begin with, she points out that *humanity* really means *male* and man defines woman as relative to him — not to herself. She is certainly not regarded as an autonomous being [9]. She states that woman "is defined and differentiated with reference to man and not he with reference to her; she is the incidental, the inessential as opposed to the essential. He is the Subject, he is the Absolute — she is the Other" [9]. These words of de Beauvoir would merely serve as inflammatory rhetoric if we did not have abundant evidence that this in fact does occur.

To begin with, earlier it was pointed out that the active character of love is *giving,* not *giving up* something or being deprived of something. Giving in this sense is a very positive and rewarding experience. It is the highest expression of potency. Certainly, over history we have rich examples of women as strong and forceful individuals because we see that they have given an abundant amount of love to their children, their husbands, their families and their friends. For most, it was an important kind of giving. It has been through this form of giving that many women have experienced a sense of strength, wealth, potency and fulfillment. To be capable of giving love to those who are significant to one is an important achievement.

If we reconsider the basic elements of love identified by Erich Fromm — care, responsibility, respect and knowledge — it is very apparent that women have indeed *given* a great deal of love. They have certainly demonstrated their concern for their families through their constant caring for them and by taking the major responsibility for meeting their basic human needs. With regard to their mates, women have given much the same kind of love.

When women have worked outside the home, they have also given generously. In the work world their giving has been comparable to the kinds of contributions they have made to their families. Also, they have made tremendous contributions to society through a vast number of volunteer organizations that provide invaluable services to people. For many women, this aspect of giving has not been viewed as a sacrifice. While it meant giving a lot of themselves, for them it was a way of giving love. They experienced a sense of fulfillment in giving. Many women today still give abundantly to their families, to organizations and to others in this way. Many women will continue to demonstrate their love for significant people in their lives by caring for them and taking responsibility for meeting human needs.

Where the problem arises, however, is when women have no choice or other options in life. When the major responsibility for child-rearing and household management is imposed upon the woman as her duty and is not equally shared by the husband, this soon turns into personal sacrifice and deprivation for the woman. When the cultural norms of society dictate through tradition and various other pressures that this is the major role for the woman with little appreciation or value for this assigned role, the woman feels devalued and exploited. Erich Fromm pointed out that responsibility could turn into possessiveness and domination if the other aspect of love — respect — is not present. When we respect others, we see, understand and appreciate their uniqueness. This respect is based on independence and freedom. Numerous examples have already been cited that illustrate the lack of independence and freedom for women. They have respected their husbands and male companions and have accepted the double standard that promotes independence and freedom for men but denies the same for women. From the beginning, women were programmed to accept and to expect to take an unequal share of responsibility in giving of themselves to others.

In regard to the aspect of love that relates to really knowing an individual, women have scored very high. They have not focused on their own concerns. Rather, they have focused their concerns on their families and have supported their needs as opposed to their own. When one considers all these facts, it is easy to see that women have been very generous and very capable in giving love to others. Unfortunately, many of these same aspects of love were not re-ciprocal. Children and husbands love them but often not in the same way. The reason is that the giving that has been expected from women has deprived them of equality, respect, freedom and a personal identity. With all her generous giving, the woman in American society is still in a position of *alterity*. She is defined by others and through others. What we see happening, then, is that the majority of women have a great capacity for giving love to others. The mature, ideal love that Fromm talks about has turned sour and lopsided for women in our society, and many are now voicing loud complaints against the injustice of the unequal and unfair expectations for them as compared to men. It is not that women no longer care to give and to love. But they are tired of being expected to give in a way that demeans them. This is not the kind of giving that Fromm was referring to. As long as any segment of society continues to pressure and program young women into believing that sacrificing and depriving themselves is the healthy, normal way of giving love, we will continue to see women who are weak. They will never become autonomous, free individuals. The women in our society who never marry or never have children are looked upon differently in relation to giving as an aspect of love. Actually, they are pitied by a vast number of people because they are first of all viewed as aberrant — and as failures. Even today, this is still true. They are often assumed to be incapable of giving or loving. Perhaps the most degrading belief is that they are unlovable. Many people do not stop to consider that there are many different kinds of love, only one of which may lead to marriage. Love directed toward friends, families or other people significant in one's life has all the same elements as the love that is labeled romantic. It is also a rewarding experience. Single women and married women both have given love abundantly in a variety of ways to many different people. One's marital status tells us little about the individual's capacity and depth in directing love to others in a meaningful way. While both single women and married women have given love generously in many different ways, to many people, groups, social institutions and organizations, they continue to be exposed to many societal expectations and pressures that prevent them from becoming autonomous, self-actualized individuals.

Both groups of women are affected in their capacity to love based on their early life experiences. I have already identified many important influences in the early socialization of girls. Since it is in this early period that the individual's self-concept is developed, one would have to agree that the socialization of a girl is a major deterrent to her sense of self-actualization. It does not seem as though most women have learned to love themselves. If they had, there would not be so many examples of women who have an undervalued self-concept. This fact seems evident, since so many women demonstrate a sense of unworthiness and are underperformers in comparison to their actual potential. Earlier, it was pointed out that people who think poorly of themselves shrink their aspirations and do not live up to their true potential. An interesting study was conducted by Matina Horner that supports this idea in relation to women. The fact that women in our society have been indoctrinated to value the traditional concepts of femininity above all else has already been discussed. Femininity, as viewed by society, is felt to be a goal incompatible with achievement. Horner conducted a study over an eight-year period which clearly demonstrated that most women have a motive in avoiding success. The college women in her study became anxious about achieving success because they expected negative consequences if they did. They felt that they would suffer social rejection and/or feelings of being unfeminine. Horner found that "women still tend to view competition, independence, intellectual achievement and leadership as basically in conflict with femininity" [10]. Women who had a high fear of success lowered their aspiration level as they progressed from their freshman to their junior year in college. For example, those who had planned on going to law school decided to teach instead. Those who wanted to be politicians planned instead to work for politicians. She concluded from her studies that higher education for women was felt to be more acceptable if the objective was to create a generally educated and therefore more interesting wife, mother and companion [10]. Another interesting finding was the high price young women are willing to pay for their anxiety about success. Many young women were found to perform at lower levels in mixed-sex competition situations. Those who did succeed often downgraded their own performance in the presence of males. Not only are the career aspirations of these women lowered and their opportunities narrowed, but many simply abdicate from competition in the outside world when faced with the conflict between their feminine image and the development of their real abilities and interests [10].

One of the most important issues pointed out in the study was the necessity to make new options available for enhancing the self-esteem of women. In the past, having children has been one of the major *acceptable* sources of this self-esteem. Since young women are now being pressured to have fewer children, their major source of self-esteem is diminishing. Since having children is another example of women developing their self-esteem through "others," the sooner this change occurs the better. If having children is one day not considered to be the most important task for a woman in life, we may find healthier, happier older women. As it is today, many older women, having fulfilled their alleged major mission in life by bearing and rearing children, feel useless, inadequate and devalued once the children leave "the nest" [10].

People who have learned to love themselves have also learned to value themselves for what they are. Because they love and value themselves, they are able to achieve success in life. Success has been defined in many ways. For our purposes here, I would like to use Jo-Ann Evans Gardner's simple definition of success: ". . . success is defined in terms of whether or not people get to do what they perceive as their work" [10]. She also states that many women have not been able to do their work. Again, the reason for this is the failure of women as a group to learn to love and value themselves, not that women are void of any degree of self-love. If they did not love themselves at all, they would be totally unable to love others. Total self-hatred by an individual often results in the self-destruction of the individual in one form or another. Individuals who have developed a strong sense of self-love approach life with a feeling of adequacy and self-confidence. They are eventually able to progress in their development until they become self-actualized individuals at first part of the time and gradually on a continuing basis.

We have all seen many examples of women who have successfully reared children and made significant contributions to the total family. There are also women, both single and married, who have used their talents, maximized their potential and have achieved success in other areas outside of the home and family. These women have been in the minority, however. Consider the many areas in which women could make significant contributions: in science, education, religion, health care, politics, industry, literature, art, journalism, television, entertainment, law, etc. Since it has been shown that girls actually excel over boys academically until approximately the high school years, and have the potential to do at least equally well at the college level, it follows that they should be capable of making important contributions in any field of interest. The fact that they do not is further evidence that the majority of women do not progress to become self-actualized.

We also know that women as a group are not autonomous. If they were, they would be self-governing and would determine their own destiny. Our history shows in part why this has not happened. For one thing, the laws of our country have held us back and kept

How Do I Love Me?

us in an inferior position. "Until fairly recently, the law treated a corporation as a person but did not recognize women except in specified circumstances" [11]. Women were the property of their fathers first and, once married, became the property of their husbands. Women could not own property, sign contracts, vote, or hold a political office. Women were incorporated and consolidated with their husbands. According to the early laws of this country, a wife did not have a separate existence from her husband. In a legal sense, she died on her wedding day. In the past, if a woman left her husband, she lost all rights to her children. The husband could also legally require his wife to submit to sexual relations against her will and to live wherever he chose [11]. To put it more succinctly, most women were legally, socially and emotionally the legitimate slaves of men in early America. Their *alterity,* or otherness, was institutionalized in all aspects of society. Some women today would argue that they are still slaves to men. Title VII of the Civil Rights Act of 1964 was amended to prohibit discrimination in employment practices on the basis of sex.* That was ten years ago. While some improvements have been made in this area, one does not have to look very far to see that women have a long way to go before they will have achieved equality in the job market. Legally and economically, women are still discriminated against. There are still married women who are professionals and earning good salaries but who cannot take out loans, make business transactions, etc., without the signature of their husbands. On the other hand, their husbands do not have to submit to the same requirements. In some instances, these women have greater job security and earn better salaries than their husbands. How can one move toward independence and autonomy when these kinds of controls are perpetuated?

When one studies the early history of women in America and the long struggle to be recognized equally under the constitution, it is no small wonder that few women today are truly autonomous.

* Howard W. Smith proposed adding the word *sex* to the amendment in a last-ditch effort to prevent passage of the law that would give black people equal access to schools, pools, accommodations and jobs. He was not really interested in equality for women. The inclusion of the word *sex* was introduced in a joking manner in an effort to block his opponents, who were determined to pass the Civil Rights Act [12].

Our society is controlled socially, economically and politically by men. Regardless of the slight inroads we may have made in these areas (they are minimal to be sure), wherever we go or whatever we do, we will be under the control of men. For the present, the only opportunity we have for autonomy is to govern our own lives on a very small scale. We are certainly capable of being responsible for our own actions and feelings. A global perspective of American society demonstrates our lack of autonomy. On a smaller scale, in our daily lives, there is also an absence of autonomy. The capacities in individuals that demonstrate autonomy are awareness, spontaneity and intimacy. At first glance, it could be said that most women have these capacities. On further evaluation, we have said that the autonomous person is aware of the world around him. His perception is based on his own experience rather than the way others taught him to perceive it. As long as women are assigned powerless roles and accept them, they can hardly be said to be autonomous. As long as others make important decisions that affect them, their perception of the world around them will be distorted and, in a sense, dictated to them. The autonomous person can be spontaneous and as such have the freedom to see many options in life. His life-style is not predetermined but is chosen on the basis of his potentialities. He consciously decides for himself what he will do because he is free. Women have certainly not had many options to chose from. Many schools, institutions, occupations and privileges have not been open to women, though recently some tokenism has occurred, and some opportunities, previously open only to men, have been made available to a small number of women. Not only do women lose autonomy through "lack of opportunities," but this is augmented by early indoctrination, socialization and tradition. Breaking away from ingrained value systems is no small task.

The last aspect of autonomy is intimacy: the expression of warmth, tenderness and closeness to others. Women certainly have been allowed, even obligated, to express intimacy — but only to a certain degree. It has been traditionally unacceptable for women to reveal too much of their intellect, too much of their deeper feelings about life, love and loved ones. Women have been taught to hide their inner selves from both other women and men and even from themselves. The socialization process taught women to deal with others on a frothy, superficial level. The only acceptable intimacy

80 was sexual, in bed with one's husband, and then one must be very careful to reveal oneself in strictly nonthreatening ways. As a result, women have been islands unto themselves — encouraged in their isolation by keeping a close check on their inner self. If women had had the freedom to reveal this inner self, their real potentials would have been recognized, respected and utilized long ago. Instead, a great deal of energy has been directed at "protecting" women (through various laws, etc.) and essentially keeping them "in their place" in the "man's world."

Another result of the historical lesser position of women in society is that they develop characteristic ways of behaving that categorize them as *losers*. They are unable to respond authentically as members of society. They avoid becoming self-responsible. Instead of learning to confront adverse situations in an aggressive, confident manner, they are forced to resort to manipulative techniques that they learned early in life. They play-act, pretend and perpetuate old roles from childhood because they have not learned to do otherwise. In fact, very often this was reinforced by those close to them. Other female role models, who behaved the same way, provided them with an identification for these stereotypic roles. Because they have not been encouraged or supported in trying new and challenging tasks, functions and roles, they have helped to perpetuate and maintain their own status quo. As a result, women over time have continued to function (with some exceptions) as their mothers did and to make the same mistakes. They have been kept in a similar dependent, powerless role, and much of their full potential has remained dormant and not utilized. There are still great numbers of women in our society today who have been so thoroughly programmed and indoctrinated about their "natural" and traditional feminine role and place in society that they defend any efforts made to maintain them. Underlying this, I believe, are a fear and anxiety about becoming autonomous. If all the influences throughout one's lifetime are primarily directed toward maintaining a predetermined role, which includes a marked state of dependency, the individual will have great difficulty in moving toward autonomy. The idea itself is frightening because of the lack of preparation for such a process and the unknown outcome.

All that I have pointed out here about the plight of women and their lack of autonomy in our society is depressing to say the least.

It is no wonder that so many women today are expressing angry feelings and resentment toward things as they are. Our situation is not hopeless, however. Many women, young and old, are beginning to recognize those forces in society that are preventing them from actualizing their full potential. They are working in a variety of ways to bring about long overdue changes. In essence, these women are learning to behave like winners. They have the positive attributes that distinguish them as winners — and they are becoming autonomous, self-actualized women. They are stimulating to be around because they know what they want to do in life, they have the necessary skills and self-confidence to achieve their goals and they are very comfortable with themselves. It is obvious that somewhere along the line they have learned to love and respect themselves. Rather than being less feminine, they seem to be more complete and autonomous human beings. Their greatest frustration is overcoming the special barriers that confront them. I am looking forward to the day when women like this will be representative of the majority and when they will not be considered rare or unusual.

Alterity of Nurses

The special problems encountered by women that pertain to love, autonomy and self-actualization are also experienced by nurses. Not only must the nurse deal with a sense of alterity in the context of society at large, but she must cope with it in a more specific way on a daily basis in the health care system. Nurses are not yet an autonomous, self-actualized group. To understand why they are not, we need to look at how nurses view themselves, how others view them and how they are defined and operate within the health care system. To begin with, nursing provides the individual practitioner with ample opportunities for loving others. Since the active character of love is giving, nurses have rich opportunities for experiencing a heightened sense of strength as they care for people. While this form of giving is hard work, it is not interpreted by most nurses as "giving up" something or being deprived of something. Quite the contrary. In a broad sense, it is a special form of love. When we provide effective and comprehensive nursing to people, all the basic elements of love are present. We are concerned and

82 therefore care for the other person. In the most significant sense, when we care for another person, we help him to grow and to actualize himself. "Through caring for certain others, by serving them through caring, a man [woman] lives the meaning of his [her] own life. In the sense in which a man [woman] can ever be said to be at home in the world, he [she] is at home not through dominating, or explaining, or appreciating, but through caring and being cared for" [13]. Because we care for and about our patients, we take responsibility for helping to meet their expressed and unexpressed needs. We do this voluntarily because this is why most of us have chosen nursing as a career — we wanted to care for others. At the same time that we take responsibility for caring for others we also respect them, for when we fail to respect the individual and his uniqueness, we dominate and depersonalize him. In order to respect the person we care for, we must first get to know him. We then learn to accept him on his own terms. If as professionals we truly care for, respect and accept the responsibility for meeting individual needs, we have an ethical responsibility to base our actions on sound and up-to-date knowledge. When optimum and comprehensive nursing is provided, these same basic elements of love as identified by Fromm will be present. In an ideal sense, then, nursing could be described as a way of giving love. The basic elements of love and the basic aspects of nursing are easily correlated. This is not in any sense an unrealistic analogy of nursing care and love. Not every nurse loves every patient and therefore meets his every need. But providing appropriate nursing care to individuals who are in need of it can be, and very often is, a form of love. For those nurses who have the capacity to provide competent, compassionate care to others, there is a sense of fulfillment just as there is in giving other forms of love. Again, as with women in general, we have abundant examples of nurses who have given a great deal of love to their patients through caring for them. Unfortunately, we also find nursing care that does not provide love and respect; it is regimented, depersonalized and inadequate.

This situation occurs because nurses, like other women, have not learned to love and value themselves. As a result, they have not become self-actualized, autonomous professional women. Their position in the health care system corresponds to the position of other women in society. One of the most important aspects of the nurse's role should be that of a "patient advocate." But she finds it difficult to function as the patient's advocate because she has little control over her own practice and destiny, is unable to function autonomously and her contributions are not significantly valued.

What proof do we have of this? The individual who does not first of all value and love himself will characteristically behave in two ways. He will not perform up to his full potential and he will demonstrate a sense of unworthiness. He will lower his aspirations to a level below his ability and depreciate himself in many ways. This negative attitude will affect all his other relationships. And so it is with many nurses.

There is plentiful evidence that nurses do not perform according to their full potential. As indicated in previous chapters, nursing education today is a rigorous process. Nursing practice is based upon theories and principles from the physical, behavioral and social sciences. The nurse, like other professionals, is expected to assess specific patient needs in a systematic and scientific manner in order to plan, implement and evaluate appropriate and effective care. Because of the bureaucratic organization of most health care settings, the nurse has become a functionary whose main contribution seems to lie in the "harnessing" process. She spends a great deal of time translating physician's orders into discrete quanta of work that are often delegated to other members of the nursing team. She also collates the many activities of the nursing staff [14]. She is expected to coordinate the plans and activities of the other health care workers who are involved with the patients' treatment program. She spends an inordinate amount of time in managing the patient care unit if she works in a hospital. In almost all settings, she has administrative responsibilities and is deluged with paperwork. Her most important skill, that of caring for patients, is frequently carried out through others with less preparation and skill. The health care settings, where most nurses are employed, are organizations with a bureaucratic type of administration for the main purpose of efficiency. When we ask "efficiency for whom?" the answer is resoundingly clear: it is to maximize organization efficiency [15]. The nurse in this system plays a supportive role that aids efficiency within the system. According to Christine Pierce, efficiency requires only that someone play the supportive role — belong to the maintenance class — and that those in this role devote their lives psychologically and physically to making sure that other people get done whatever they want done [16]. In this situation, the nurse plays a supportive role to the administrator, the physician and sometimes other health care professionals. This, of course, contributes efficiency to the very power structure that prevents nurses from developing freedom in their own role choices and functions. In the past, it was common knowledge that slaves played a very supportive role for their masters, and of course society was more efficient and comfortable because of this. The price was "freedom" [16]. Nurses too are paying a very high price for their supportive role. They lack freedom and autonomy.

There are other examples of nurses not utilizing or actualizing their full potential. The nurse has frequent and immediate contact with patients and therefore makes important observations. If it were not for these observations, the physician often would be unable to make significant interpretations and to initiate appropriate action. Though much of what the physician bases his decisions on are observations and findings reported by the nurse, she is often not credited with this. The nurse also has the scientific background which enables her to use judgment in making independent decisions as necessary and appropriate. Unfortunately, many times her knowledge and her interpretations are regarded as less valid and are less apt to be given credence than those of the physician. It is sad to admit, but many nurses share this view of themselves. Katz has pointed out that the crucial point here is not "Who knows the most?" but rather "Who is the *rightful* knower?" Both the physician and the nurse acknowledge and accept the physician as the ultimate guardian of knowledge about the patient's illness or condition. He also points out that physicians are often apt to have knowledge about the patient that is not available to the nurse, and Katz suggests that this has helped to lower the nurse's status [14]. It is incredible to me that this still frequently occurs in all types of health care settings. The issue is not who is better educated, the physician or the nurse. Rather, it is that their education is comparable yet different in many ways — and his knowledge is recognized while hers is not.

Many nurses, when they do have specific knowledge about patients, still refuse to give out any information regarding their condition, their vital signs, their medications, etc., even when requested to do so by the patient. This is one of the most common examples of nurses either not being allowed (because of hospital policy or individual physician's idiosyncrasies) to use their own initiative and professional judgment or simply refusing because they were taught not to divulge information.

All patients have the right to know what their physical condition is, what treatment is planned for them, what risks are involved, and what outcomes are expected. In most states, it is now a law that all medications prescribed must have the name and dosage clearly marked on the label. Unless there are very special or extraordinary reasons why a patient should not be given certain information, I feel it is the nurse's professional and ethical responsibility to be honest and informative with him. I would hope that more nurses will consider their responsibility for health-teaching and will take the initiative to inform their patients adequately and fairly.

Recently a friend of mine (who is not a nurse) had a harrowing experience in a hospital where her critically ill mother was being cared for after suffering several strokes. These strokes had affected her mother's ability to communicate, and she was frightened and confused about what was happening to her. She had always been a strong, self-directing woman, and her inability to speak or to care for herself was embarrassing and anxiety producing. Because of this, it was difficult for her to express to the nursing staff or physician the many questions and concerns that she had. Because she was comfortable and more relaxed with her family, she was able to communicate more effectively with them. Also, they took the time to understand her attempts at speaking. She asked them questions about her condition, what medications and treatments she was being given and why and what to expect in the future. The physician in this situation had not given the patient or the family any of this information. When the nurses came to give her medication or to carry out some procedure, my friend would attempt to find out what they were doing and why. The nurses refused to tell her and instead referred her to the physician, thus passing up many opportunities for doing health-teaching with the patient and her family. Not only would it have helped prepare her for when she went home, but it would also have eliminated a great deal of stress and anxiety for both the patient and her family.

Another example that illustrates the nurse's "underperformance" is in the area of judgment and decision-making. All of us were taught to "carry out doctor's orders." Now according to the Nurse Practice Acts in most states, this is a legal requirement for the nurse. I would like to add here, however, that some of those orders are ridiculous and should not go unchallenged. In fact, as a professional, the nurse also has a legal responsibility to question and to refuse to carry out an order that would seem to jeopardize the health or safety of a patient. Many physicians I know do not seem to understand or acknowledge this fact. Most nurses are conscientious about carrying out appropriate physician orders. They do not often enough, however, make independent decisions based on their own judgment, which has frequently been shown to be very sound. For example, accompanying patients when they are admitted to the hospital is their medical record, which sometimes contains pages of physician's orders. Many of these orders are for quite routine procedures, and of course many are specific to the health problem of the patient. Many times, the physician routinely orders that the vital signs be taken a specified number of times during the day. This may be important initially because it may contribute information that relates to identifying the patient's specific health problem or response to treatment. Repeatedly it happens that the patient's vital signs continue to be taken, sometimes until he leaves, when it is no longer necessary. If they are taken around the clock, this means the patient will be awakened at night unnecessarily, and unless the doctor remembers to discontinue this order or unless someone reminds him to do so, this continues. Certainly in this situation and many others, a competent nurse should be able to make the decision to discontinue this task. This is only one example of how nurses' skill and judgment in a clinical situation are not properly utilized. Dozens more could be cited.

The fact that many nurses continue to function without questioning orders is further evidence of how thoroughly they have been indoctrinated into a dependent, subservient role. A factor that contributes to this is the doctor-nurse "game" they are expected to play. Doctors give and write "orders." They order others to perform specific functions. Nurses merely "suggest." Their suggestions have to be presented to the physician in such a way as to appear not to be telling him what to do. For instance, the nurse does not usually say (based on her observations and experience),

"John Jones is having a lot of pain and the Darvon is not relieving him.
I think he needs Demerol." That would irritate most physicians and
the nurse would be considered "out of line." Instead, she is more likely
to say "John Jones is still having a lot of pain and the Darvon does not
seem to relieve him. Could he perhaps have something stronger — like
Demerol?" In this situation, she has played the game according to the
proper rules. She has merely raised a question or suggested a change.
Frequently, the physician will honor the request of the nurse (if it is
addressed to him in the proper manner) and will dutifully write an
"order" which she can then carry out. The fact that it was through her
observation and judgment that the treatment regimen was changed will
not be acknowledged. If the change she suggested is effective, that will
usually not be acknowledged either. If, on the other hand, she makes an
error in some aspect of the patient's treatment, this will definitely be
acknowledged. She will, like a child, be scolded by the physician, often
in front of many other people, and she may be admonished by someone
else in the nursing hierarchy. Situations like these could be reported by
thousands of nurses. It does not take the nurse long, in any setting, to
figure out what the ground rules are that will dictate her role and
function. To function as an autonomous, professional woman, she
has to be willing to take on the whole system. For those few who have
tried, it is an overwhelming task. They have not often succeeded
either, because they lack support from just about everyone in the
system, including other nurses.

When individuals are forced to lower their aspirations continually and
to use only a portion of their real potential, they come to depreciate themselves. They develop a sense of unworthiness and they then behave in
characteristic ways. If we look at nurses as a group, we can see multiple
examples of self-depreciation. At first glance, it might appear that nurses
are merely humble or modest. On closer examination, however, it becomes
obvious that they have low self-esteem. To begin with, there is a rather
rigid social stratification system in most health care settings. Within this
formalized system, physicians are placed at the top in castelike super-
ordination above nurses. Nurses, along with many other health care professionals, are not located on a continuum with physicians. The caste-like
system has placed an unscalable wall between the other health care professionals and the physician [14]. Within this system the nurse "knows
her place." Her place, even today, is still a subservient, subordinate one.
The nurse behaves accordingly: she accepts the knowledge domain as

that of the physician, so she maintains her silence with patients. She does not trespass by giving patients information about themselves when she has the knowledge to do so. Modern medicine has prestige because it rests on recognized scientific principles. It has received great public acclaim because of the scientific and technological advances that have been made in treating illness. Nursing does not share in this prestige, and nursing care is not viewed by the public as necessarily based on scientific principles. Instead, nurses are viewed as assistants to physicians, who are the real guardians and promoters of scientific medicine. Nurses assist them in many specific ways but as distinct underlings who simply follow instructions. Nurses are not accepted as part of the scientific fraternity that exists in health care settings. They are disfranchised from equal participation and are separate from physicians. For the most part, nurses have accepted their low status and position, so it would seem reasonable to conclude that their self-esteem is not very high. Many believe this is the way things should be. Katz found that physicians hold nurses in low esteem as well. He states that while physicians often acknowledge competence and fondness for individual nurses, they are still willing to see nurses receive infinitely smaller incomes than their own and often treat the nurse as a "nonperson" [14]. Again an analogy can be made between specific black slaves and their masters. Some were liked and treated kindly, but they were expected to "stay in their place."

In June 1974, the California Nurses' Association represented 4,000 nurses in northern California in their strike actions against three private hospital groups. The major issues included demands by nurses for staffing of adequately prepared personnel in specialized units (such as intensive care units), more control over staffing patterns for nurses, every other weekend scheduled off, adequate portable pension plan and establishment of health insurance and other benefits for part-time nurses. The nurses also asked for increases in salary to keep up with inflation. None of these demands was unreasonable. In fact, the concern the nurses shared regarding proper education of personnel who were assigned to specialty units was certainly in the best interest of better and safer patient care. The practice that was occurring in the hospitals involved was anything but safe. When short-staffing occurred in one of the specialty units and no other help could be found, nurses and other nursing staff were "pulled" from other patient care areas to "fill in." These individuals often did not have the expertise or knowledge to care adequately or safely for the critically ill patients in these units. When the hospital representatives refused to meet the requests of the nurses, the nurses went on strike. They did not take this action irresponsibly or without a great deal of prior planning. They set up a staffing committee to evaluate critical care nursing needs and to fill those needs during the strike. The strike took place while the American Nurses' Convention met in San Francisco. The commentators on the local television news programs were fair in their presentation of the problems and the progress in the negotiations that were going on. The public support regarding the nurses' actions was gratifying. Everywhere, taxi drivers, waiters and waitresses, business operators, hotel staff and people on the street expressed their approval of the strike. A representative of the American Medical Association, however, adamantly stated "patient care is the responsibility of the physician — not the nurse!" He went on to criticize the striking nurses for their inappropriate concern and behavior and charged that nurses were neglecting patients and jeopardizing patients' health by striking. This of course was not the case. He was appearing on a national news program as the official voice speaking on behalf of the physicians in this country. While some physicians may not have agreed and may have been supportive of the nurses' action, the powerful A.M.A. spoke officially for physicians in this country, and its stand on this issue tells us a great deal about their opinion of nursing. It tells us even more about their philosophy, their sense of power and their need to control others in the health care system.

About a year after this incident, a group of resident physicians in several hospitals in New York (and later on in California) were dissatisfied with the quality of patient care and their own working conditions and threatened to strike. Counterthreats were made by hospital representatives. These included firing physicians who walked off their jobs. Support from nurses was voiced loud and clear. Many indicated they would also leave in support of the physicians' actions. When I read newspaper accounts of the issues raised by these physicians, I agreed with their action. They too were concerned about patient care and were unable to convince hospital representatives to make necessary changes. Only withdrawal of their needed services drew attention to their dilemma. The American Nurses' Association did not appear on a national telecast to berate these physicians for their action. Many nurses were willing to jeopardize their jobs to support their physician co-workers. Nurses who have collectively organized to improve patient care, their work environment, their fringe benefits, their salaries or their power in decision-making have not been well-supported by physicians. On the other hand, nurses have been quick to support physicians when they have done the same thing.

As we can see, the plight of most nurses is not really so different from women in general. Only the stage and the actors are different.

Why are nurses loyal and cooperative in health care settings when their esteem is obviously so low? Katz suggests that nurses accept partial payment for the slights they endure by being "permitted" to carry out nurturant care functions that really have no clear place in modern medicine. "It is as though the nurse receives the right to engage in her traditional tasks as a bonus for accepting second-class citizenship in the dominant medical system. The system benefits from this arrangement, since nurturant care of some sort is doubtless essential for most patients" [14]. I am happy to report that cracks are now beginning to appear in the caste system as many of the "new breed" young nurses enter the system with a different attitude and more self-confidence. Many young people today are unwilling to accept the old authoritarian model of dictatorship. They expect at least respect for their ideas and will not accept things as they are merely because of tradition. Some consumers are getting in on the act also and are beginning to demand their rights as patients. Together, these groups may peel away some of the mystique within the health system and eventually get to the core of the "pathological" organization within the system.

Another area that demonstrates low status and esteem for nurses is the economic compensation for giving "tender loving care." TLC for the most part is paid for "in the non-negotiable currency of temporary pleasant feelings, not in social recognition that takes the form of a respectable wage" [14]. The lesser value placed on care as compared to cure has already been discussed. Again, TLC is women's work and therefore not as valued.

When one considers the time and energy involved in the educational process of a nurse, it is an abomination that her potential is underutilized; she is kept from developing a true sense of autonomy as a professional women. As long as the male-dominated, physician-dominated, castelike health care system is perpetuated and sustained, the talents and potentials of nurses will be wasted. Nurses will continue to appear as losers; they will remain dependent, and their role and function will continue to be defined by others. They will not be self-actualized and will therefore be unable to deal effectively with the multiple problems in the complex health care system. Traditional, stereotypic roles left over from earlier times in nursing will be perpetuated and reinforced. Many of the mistakes from our past will be repeated because individuals will not have the courage to try new things. Individual talent and intellect will be wasted, which is a terrible price to pay.

As women and nurses we must become winners. It is not easy to become and remain a winner. "It takes courage to experience the freedom that comes with autonomy, courage to accept intimacy and directly encounter other persons, courage to take a stand in an unpopular cause, courage to choose authenticity over approval and to choose it again and again, courage to accept the responsibility for your own choices, and indeed, courage to be the very unique person you really are" [8].

Nurses, and women in society at large, are strong human beings. They have demonstrated tremendous capacities for loving. They also have a need to be loved. When they begin to love and value themselves more, and when others love, value and accept them on an equal basis, they will develop the courage that it takes to become a winner. They will become more autonomous and self-actualized. And then our society will be a better place in which to live.

References

1. Munro, Eleanor. *Viva Victoria*. *Ms.,* Vol. III, No. 7, January 1975, p. 101.
2. Fromme, Allan. *The Ability to Love*. New York: Pocket Books, 1974, p. 16.
3. Fromm, Erich. *The Art of Loving*. New York: Harper & Row, 1956, p. 17.
4. Coppersmith, Stanley. *The Antecedents of Self-Esteem*. San Francisco: Freeman, 1967, pp. 4–5.
5. Dinkmeyer, Don. *Child Development – The Emerging Self*. Englewood Cliffs, N.J.: Prentice-Hall, 1965, pp. 183–184.
6. Maslow, Abraham. *Toward a Psychology of Being*. New York: Van Nostrand, 1968.

92   7. Ibid., p. 97.

8. James, Muriel, and Jongeward, Dorothy. *Born to Win: Transactional Analysis with Gestalt Experiments.* Reading, Mass.: Addison-Wesley, 1973.

9. de Beauvoir, Simone. *The Second Sex.* New York: Vintage Books, 1974.

10. Horner, Matina, and Walsh, Mary. Psychological Barriers to Success in Women. In *Women and Success: The Anatomy of Achievement,* Kundsin, Ruth (Ed.). New York: William Morrow, 1974.

11. Bird, Caroline. *Born Female.* New York: Pocket Books, 1974.

12. Ibid., pp. 1—4.

13. Mayeroff, Milton. *On Caring,* Anshen, Ruth Nanda (Ed.). New York: Harper & Row, 1971.

14. Katz, Fred E. Nurses. In *The Semi Professions and Their Organization,* Etzioni, Amitai (Ed.). New York: Free Press, 1969.

15. Blau, Peter. *Bureaucracy in Modern Society.* New York: Random House, 1968.

16. Pierce, Christine. Natural Law Language and Women. In *Woman in Sexist Society: Studies in Power and Powerlessness,* Gornick, Vivian. and Moran, Barbara (Eds.). New York: Basic Books, 1971.

4   Other Women

Carol Spengler

*The odd thing about these deep
and personal connections of
women is that they often ignore
barriers of age, economics,
worldly experience, race,
culture — all the barriers that,
in male or mixed society, had
seemed so difficult to cross [1].*
Gloria Steinem

Women as individuals and as a group need to change, to flourish, to grow to a point where they have a sense of completeness based on an inner feeling of self-love and respect. Not only must women learn to love themselves but they must learn to love, value, trust and respect other women. Since the women's movement began in the early sixties, many women have learned to do this. And they have found enormous rewards as they have developed a sense of *sisterhood* and relatedness with other women. There is no doubt that we are making important progress in this area. The fact that many women are still isolated from each other indicates that we have a great deal of work to do. The privatism or isolation of women continues in many ways that are both subtle and obvious. One could argue that this is not true because women have always had other women friends. And they have, to be sure. If we look beyond the surface and consider how women have traditionally related to one another, we gain an important perspective. We can understand better why women *seem* to be close to one another but are still too often uncomfortable and mistrustful of other women.

To begin with, we can observe women in many different situations and note that there are pairs and groups of women together almost everywhere. We see women shopping together, lunching together, talking together, working together, laughing together, living together and doing a dozen other things together. But how do they really feel about each other? How much do they trust one another and what are the limits to this? Why are they together? Do women value other women? Do they truly become friends?

Women's Relationships with Each Other

Feminists for some time now have attempted to increase our awareness of the common or usual characteristics of women's relationships with one another. To begin with, there are many traits that women have in common. Phyllis Chesler describes these traits as naivete, self-hatred, reproductive narcissism, compulsive heterosexuality, masochism, distrust of other women along with idealism, compassion and passion [2]. Since all but a few of these traits could easily be classified as negative characteristics, one could argue that there seems to be no sound reason for women to get together. Yet they do get together.

On Friendship

Many women would tell you that it is for "friendship or social" reasons that they spend time together. Most people would readily say that they understand the meaning of friendship. Because friendship is integral to our well-being, however, let us purposely examine the variety of definitions of friendship. The word *friend* or *friendship* usually implies a form of love. A friend is a cherished, significant person who can be trusted to share intimate thoughts and feelings. In a friendship, there is a sense of attachment, affection and esteem. In short, the basic elements of love are present in the relationship. Friends care for one another, take some responsibility for one another, respect each other and know and understand each other in a special way. Friends trust each other; each knows the other's vulnerabilities. They do not exploit one another. They do not dominate one another. They see the strengths and weaknesses in one another; they enjoy and appreciate the strengths and give encouragement and support to change the weaknesses if that is desired. Friends often share common interests. When friendship exists between two people, each has the feeling "I like you because you're you." It's a comfortable relationship because each person can be herself — each knows that "being myself" is accepted and even valued.

Friends can be quite different from one another in many ways and yet value those differences in each other. All human beings have the capacity to establish friendships. In fact, all of us — men and women — have a basic need to have friends. Sometimes our friends are of the same sex and sometimes not. The important thing is that we feel close to our friends, we share with them and we trust them. If these aspects of the relationship are not present, we classify the other person as an acquaintance.

In light of these ideas, do most women develop relationships with other women that could be labeled friendship? Many women today, through a variety of means, are discovering the rewards and the sense of closeness in developing friendships with other women. They have become more fully aware of the uniqueness and value in individual women. As they open up to each other and share their common experiences as women (whatever they might be), they are finding that they no longer feel isolated. They are able to relate to one another in a positive, supportive way. They are becoming friends. The literature is replete with testimonials that support this. The women who are having these experiences are very fortunate. Perhaps it is the first time in history that so large a number of women have learned to value the friendship of other women. There are still a great number of women, however, who demonstrate their feelings about other women through characteristic behavior. They respond and relate to other women politely, cautiously, superficially or competitively. In a sense, this response is understandable. It begins with their own self-esteem. If women have not learned to love and value themselves, it stands to reason that the person who is similar to them will also not be loved and valued. Because of this, many women do not learn to trust each other. Other women are a threat. They therefore learn to relate to their "natural" enemy (the other woman) in a superficial or competitive way. This superficiality and lack of trust is perpetuated by generation after generation of women. It is somehow part of a subtle process that goes on along with all of the other socializing forces in a woman's life

Other Women

span. It is the greatest enemy of sisterhood and friendship among women. The common characteristics that are identifiable in many relationships between women illustrate these ideas.

On Conformists
Women as a group have tended to be conformists. As little girls, they learned to conform to adult demands much more readily than little boys. Throughout their socialization, conformity to traditional feminine behavior was reinforced. Of course, males are expected to conform also. The difference is that conformity for the ideal male usually implies conformity to action, mobility, thought, struggle and pleasure. For the female, conformity usually implies conforming to inaction, emotionality, resignation and un-happiness [2]. As adults, then, women are well-prepared for main-taining the status quo of traditional femininity. Differences among women are not well tolerated. There seems almost to be a sense of terror or threat when differences among women are noted. As a result, women "police" other women [2]. They critically observe how other women behave, dress, relate to others, etc. This policing takes place within various groups and within the family structure. It begins with the mother initiating her daughter into the traditional feminine role. The daughter will do likewise with her daughter. When any of these women rebels against her "natural" role, she will be ridiculed and treated harshly, in one way or another, by other women. The punishment that women receive from other women for daring to be different often reveals a personal viciousness that is not equaled among male groups [3]. The woman who fails to imitate and emulate those characteristic behaviors and attitudes that reflect the feminine ideal will be "put down" by other women. The method may be polite but direct, or it may be cutting and dis-respectful. It may be subtle (and cruel) and may isolate the woman who dares to be different, and she may be ignored. Regardless of the method used, the woman clearly gets the picture that she is not complying with acceptable standards for feminine behavior. Because so many women have a low sense of self-esteem, they fall into the trap of conforming. The habit that women have of being critical of one another and putting each other down is the major barrier to developing a sense of togetherness and relatedness. It makes us our own worst enemies.

Chesler has pointed out that the policing phenomenon that occurs among women is rooted in the anguish of powerlessness [2]. While women lack power and control over much of their lives, they can exercise their sense of power by controlling the typical behavior of those who are in their same position — that is, other women. What many women have not stopped to consider is that the real control for maintaining the female status quo rests with the males in our society, for it is they who control society. Women's policing of other women is a means for keeping women in their place. When women are encouraged to behave as they please and are given equal opportunities, they are a threat to the status quo of the larger society. Any group that has power will seek to maintain that power. Power is not something that is easily given up. Black people discovered this when they attempted to obtain their freedom. It was a long, hard struggle up from slavery, and the struggle continues today. There were black people along the way who stood in the way of progress and equality for blacks. They were afraid to challenge the status quo. Women who police other women are also standing in the way of equality and progress because they too are afraid to challenge the status quo. The consciousness-raising groups that have sprung up all over the country are beginning to break down some of the barriers among women. As a result, some women are not conforming to the usual pressures and are discovering instead that it is exciting and rewarding to be different.

On Competitiveness
Another common characteristic that can be seen in women's relationships with one another is competitiveness. Women compete with one another in a variety of ways. Competing, as it has come to be known in America, usually involves contending with others in some way for a prize. The prize may be as simple as being declared the winner over others. Competition is synonymous with rivalry. Frequently, where women are concerned, competition revolves around men. This occurs in several ways. Women learn early in life to value themselves as they are desired by others. As youngsters, their affirmation of desirability is dependent on their parents and other people significant to them. When they become adults, their male partner becomes their source of affirmation [4].

100 Since women's success is still defined in relation to their ability to establish a relationship with a man and eventually to marry, there is a great deal of competition among women in this area. The man, then, becomes the prize, and it's every woman for herself. Other women are viewed as rivals — as the enemy, so to speak. Once the woman has established a relationship with her male companion, her competition with other women does not stop. Other women are always viewed as a possible threat to her security. Because of this, the woman clearly establishes "her territory" with other women. This drama is played out every day in a variety of ways. For example, in a social setting with both sexes represented, the woman who lingers too long in her conversations with another woman's husband or companion will be suspect because she poses a threat, the threat being that the "other woman" might be found more attractive, more interesting, more intelligent — more "anything" than she herself is. Women deal with this threat in different ways. Some women carefully keep track of the situation and move discreetly into closer proximity to the male and reestablish their territory. Others make left-handed compliments, remarking that they can always count on their husband to find an attractive woman to talk to. This is intended to give the husband the message, of course, that he has been noticed talking to another woman, and it tells the other woman that she is in dangerous territory. Another way to deal with the "other woman" is to criticize her to the male involved. Direct confrontation with the woman who poses a threat occurs at times also. Very often, when a woman loses a man to another woman, it is not the man who is despised but the other woman. This happens over and over again. Both women adore the man and would suffer great consequences to have him or his attention. Each woman sees the other as the person at fault in the situation. The man is fortunate in that he can choose between either woman — and in some cases opts for both.

Women have not had the same opportunities as men to compete in more constructive ways. For example, men have had many opportunities to compete with others through sports, politics, jobs, the arts, entertainment, etc. This has encouraged men to develop their skills and talents in many areas, while women are forced to compete with one another *through* others. They compete with other women on the basis of their husband's status, their family's reputation or position, their children's grades or accomplishments, etc. Men, it seems, compete with one another on the basis of their own merits. It is one thing to be proud of those you love or admire, but this is not the same as basing one's own sense of worth and identity on the position and achievements of others. This is demoralizing.

Women also compete with each other on the basis of their physical appearance or achievement as related to traditional feminine tasks. Often, when women socialize with each other, they compare themselves on the basis of attractiveness. Some of the thoughts that run through their minds as they size up another woman are that the other woman is prettier, that she is thinner, that her dress is newer or more expensive, or that her hair is more stylish. Comparisons regarding feminine tasks involve cooking, happy or healthy children, housekeeping or thrift. Women may "score" themselves in relation to other women in a positive or negative way. A great deal depends on their self-concept and their particular value system.

The important point to be made about the competition that occurs between women is that it serves as a barrier which prevents women from seeing the value in each other as individuals. Their self-esteem continues to be rooted in pleasing and living through others. This influences women to relate to one another in a superficial and skeptical manner.

On Motivation and Success
Women's motivation to avoid success is another characteristic which influences their relationships with one another. Basically, women are afraid of success in other than traditional feminine roles. Success in a profession or occupation is considered by both sexes to be deviant behavior for women [5]. As a result, many women experience a high degree of anxiety and fear in relation to success in a career. This could be explained in part "because women's success is in such short supply, and, as with all scarce commodities that we value, we worry about wanting it, feel guilty about having it, and don't quite know how to cope with it when we get it" [6]. Because successful women are viewed by many as abnormal, several outcomes have developed which interfere with female relationships.

First of all, these women are viewed as a threat to other women and to men. They are different from the majority of other women.

102 As a result, they have less in common with them and therefore have less support and less acceptance. In some ways, they could be viewed as more isolated from other women than the women who follow a more traditional pattern of functioning. To be successful, they have had to meet higher standards than most men in their same field. Among their female peers, they rarely find support [7]. What happens to these women and how do they react to this situation? Some women who achieve success in the work world think of themselves as different. Because they are different, they do not want to associate with their own group. They want to identify up, not down [3]. Therefore, they identify with men. What may eventually develop in some women is the Queen Bee syndrome. The Queen Bee is a woman who has scrapped her way up in the man's world. Interestingly, she tacitly joins with women who have been successful in traditional feminine roles to oppose the aims of feminism. All social revolutions begin with a group of militants who organize and fight for a common goal. They are soon followed by a vocal group of countermilitants who organize and fight to maintain the status quo. This has occurred with the women's liberation movement. We now have feminists and antifeminists. Some of the people who could be described as antifeminists have the characteristics of people who are against most forms of social change. The other antifeminists are called Queen Bees. They have their roots of personal success within the system where they have achieved success. This includes their professional success (which means a well-paying job with high status) as well as their social success (which means attractiveness, popularity with men, and a good marriage). "The true Queen Bee has made it in the 'man's world' of work, while running a house and family with her left hand" [8]. Her attitude is that she helped herself without the help of the women's movement and other women can too if they want to.

In the work world, several things happen in relation to Queen Bees. First of all, newcomers in an organization that has previously been exclusive (usually male) agree to be unthreatening and cooperative in exchange for advancement, benefits and praise. Second, they enjoy a privileged position not available to the majority of their peer group. Queen Bees enjoy being "rare and special." The fact that they are not to "rock the boat" is of no great concern. Their special position is. They do not relish competition for their job any more than most men do. They have **103** typically worked very hard to obtain their special position. Since their own initiation was difficult, they do not want it to be any easier for younger women than it was for them. They work to exclude any competition. They make no effort to help other women — they are too much of a threat, and Queen Bees have too much at stake. They are rewarded highly for "thinking like a man and looking so feminine." Because of the rewards they receive, they do not feel animosity toward the system or the men in the system. They identify with their male colleagues rather than with women. They reject the ideas of current feminist thinking and blame women themselves for their status as second-class citizens. They have achieved success as an individual, not as a member of a group. The attainment of success as individuals allows them to enhance their self-esteem considerably. The Queen Bee is different from feminists in several ways. She supports individualism, chooses personal goals and believes in individual strategies. Feminists, on the other hand, work as a collective toward political goals using group strategies. It is interesting to note that while Queen Bees see themselves as different from other women and do not identify with them, they share a similar ideology with women who are successful in the traditional feminine role. Both view the women's movement as a threat to their social and personal success. Both groups have been rewarded for playing a traditional role [9]. The fact that these two groups of women share the common goal of maintaining the status quo in regard to women does not mean that these groups relate to each other. Other women are still viewed as a threat to both groups. They will do little to work toward equality for the rest of the women who are concerned about the rights of women. Certainly, there are successful women who do not develop the Queen Bee syndrome. These women are sensitive and helpful to other women who are struggling to achieve success themselves. Successful women who take the time to look back and to assist other women are those who truly understand the meaning of friendship. Friendship for them can take place in their work world or in their social setting. The success experienced by another woman does not devalue or discredit their own success. They value themselves and can therefore appreciate and enjoy the success of others. We need more women like this. They are our best role models.

In summary, women's relationships with one another in many instances are characterized by a sense of isolation; lack of group cohesiveness; pressure to conform to traditonal behaviors through policing activities; competitiveness from a lack of trust; fear of success; lack of support for other women when success is experienced in other than the traditional feminine role.

Nurses' Relationships with Each Other

When comparing nurses with the greater female population, similar patterns are observable regarding their relationships with one another. While nurses share some common interests and are closely linked in the work situation, many have not developed a sense of sisterhood and relatedness with their peers. In fact, all the aspects that tend to characterize women's relationships with one another also hold true among nurses. Isolationism, lack of group cohesiveness, conformity, fear of success and competitiveness are as apparent in the nursing profession as in other groups of women.

On Isolationism versus Group Action

The isolationism that occurs in nursing is primarily because of a lack of group cohesiveness. When a group of individuals, such as nurses, who have a number of common concerns do not form a cohesive group, the individual members lack a sense of support. They feel isolated and alone in attempting to solve problems related to their specific work situation. Changes of any significant magnitude are usually brought about by groups that work collectively toward a common goal. The energy and power generated from a group effort are naturally much greater and therefore more apt to be successful in attaining a goal than is the effort of one lone individual. It seems that in nursing we are able to nurture, protect and foster growth in everyone but other nurses. Just like other women, we seem to take care of everyone else. We take care of the physician, other health care professionals, the health care system when others are not available (i.e., at night, on weekends, etc.) and patients (in the remaining time). We are so busy taking care of others that we do not take care of ourselves and other nurses. We do not organize our efforts together often enough. This is a pervasive problem in nursing at every level: at the local level within

the health care agency, at the community level, at the state level, at
the national level. It is not that nurses lack formal, organized structures
to work within. In most health care agencies, there is an organized department of nursing. If nurses would learn to talk to each other and to
sit down together to identify their mutual problems, they could form a
cohesive, powerful group. In areas where nurses have done this, they
have practically moved mountains. Together they have fought hard for
improved standards of practice, improved working conditions, improved
salaries — and perhaps most important, improved self-esteem and respect.
That this *is* occurring with greater regularity among groups of nurses is
evidence that at least some nurses are learning to share and communicate
with one another in more effective ways. They are learning to value each
other as women. Still, the large majority of nurses would tell us
that they do not feel that their problems are understood or supported by either their peers or nursing administrators. This sense of
isolation immobilizes them and prevents them from taking aggressive
action in solving the problems they experience in the work setting.
Sometimes, this lack of support seems rampant throughout the
entire nursing department. It reaches all the way to the director
or dean of nursing, who may be unable to provide the kind of leadership needed because she lacks support from the administration.

At the community level, nurses seldom form working groups
with other nurses. As a result, each group of nurses struggles
separately with common issues or concerns. Instead of maximizing the energy directed toward problem-solving, a great deal of
extra effort is expended with little or no resolution of common
problems. For example, continuing education programs are vital
to all nurses to update their knowledge and skills in their related
area of practice. All health care agencies have some responsibility
in providing educational opportunities for their professional staff.
This is an established standard for accreditation of agencies. In
order to meet this need in an effective, efficient and economical
way, programs could be organized by groups of agencies in the area
that offer similar services. This kind of sharing could result in
savings for all concerned, in time, effort and money. This does not
happen to any appreciable degree because nurses, even in smaller
areas, remain isolated from one another.

On a statewide basis, there is a wide variety of opportunities
for nurses to form collectives to meet common goals. The most

obvious is the state nurses' association. When an individual nurse joins the American Nurses' Association, she automatically becomes a member of the state and district association. Since less than one-third of all nurses belong to their professional association, the potential for strong collective action is weakened. Many state associations lack vitality, energy and leadership. In associations that enjoy these characteristics, there is a unity among nurses that enables them to zero in on significant issues that pertain to nursing and health care.

A situation that occurred in Massachusetts not long ago is a prime example. The governor, in his efforts to reorganize the state Department of Human Services, proposed to abolish the Board of Registration in Nursing as a separate agency. The functions of this board would have been assigned to a Health System Regulation Administration in the Department of Human Services. Rules and regulations regarding education and licensure that govern nursing and other health professions would have been established by a Health Systems Regulation Council. Provisions included in the proposal would have allowed *anyone* employed in a licensed or approved health care facility to perform *any* nursing tasks. In essence, this would have removed mandatory licensure for nurses, and the public would not have been properly protected from unqualified and/or unsafe practitioners. Under this proposal, Massachusetts would not have been allowed to use State Board Test Pool examinations for registered and practical nurses, since only boards of nursing are allowed to contract for these. Graduates would have been able to practice in the state without a license, but they would not have been able to practice in any other state. Their mobility would therefore have been limited. Nurses from the two professional organizations, the Practical Nurses' Association and the Student Nurse Association, collectively organized, marched on the capitol and demanded that the governor's proposal be rescinded [10]. And the nurses won! It was only through the efforts of many nurses, who were organized and unified in their strategies, that the decision was changed. One person alone or a group divided could not have accomplished this political feat.

There are many other areas within individual states that nurses could become involved in if they would pool and organize their talents. They could then form pressure groups to communicate with state organizations, state health agencies and any other institutions or groups that make decisions which affect nursing and health care.

On a national level, there is perhaps even less cohesion. For one thing, many nurses feel removed from those activities and issues that do not affect them on a daily basis. For example, the debates that are taking place in Congress regarding National Health Insurance are viewed by many nurses as an issue that has little relevance for them. If they would only consider the issue from the standpoint of being a consumer like everyone else, they would see the relevance of attempting to understand the implications of this legislation. As health care providers, nurses should study and evaluate the significance and impact of this legislation on the system of health care. More importantly, they should demand a significant role and greater recognition in any legislation involved in health care services. On this one issue alone, individual nurses can do little by themselves other than write their congressman (and a few congresswomen). As a collective group, they can support many strategies for action with a much greater chance for success.

We recently experienced success on a national level when nurses (through the two professional associations) joined with other groups to push Congress to override the President's veto on a two-year health services authorization bill. Included in this law are measures that authorize the extension of the Nurse Training Act, the National Health Service Corps, and such health service programs as family planning, public health formula grants, community mental health centers, migrant health centers and rodent control. This law authorizes 553 million dollars for loans and scholarships for nursing students as well as grants for construction of nursing school facilities. Many nurses all over the country responded to the requests of the professional organizations to become involved and to take initiative in promoting the enactment of this legislation. Without the support of nurses at the grass-roots level, this important legislation would not have survived. Certainly a greater number of nurses are banding together at all levels to work toward mutual goals. Those nurses who are involved together do not experience the isolation, loneliness and frustration that other nurses do. From my own experience, I still observe a large number of nurses who face many frustrating problems at work daily. They complain

108 about their plight to other nurses and find consensus among their peers about their frustrations. This consensus often breaks down, however, when it comes time to develop some problem-solving and to devise strategies. Support and cohesion are lacking, and the nurses' sense of isolation is deepened. These professional women, lacking cohesion and support among themselves, are therefore comparable to women in general.

On Conformity

Another characteristic that typifies nurses' relationships with one another is that of conformity. Nursing, as a female-intensive profession, in many ways epitomizes characteristic conforming behavior. We, too, have a policing system in operation. Differences among nurses are frequently no better tolerated than differences among other women. Nurses critically observe other nurses in relation to how they behave, function in their role, relate to others, etc. Differences in individual nurses seem to bring about a sense of threat to other nurses just as with other women. Policing occurs in many ways within the nursing profession beginning very early in the professional life of the nurse.

The reinforcement of acceptable feminine behavior is already operant in the individual when she enters her educational program. The pre-nursing socialization, firmly entrenched, is reinforced when the individual becomes a student. Many of the Victorian, sexist attitudes of the past continue to be perpetuated in schools of nursing. These attitudes are demonstrated through specific behaviors. In the past, instructors used to measure hemlines to ensure that they were the "proper," required length — not too short, that is. This is no longer done. Instead, we now measure the student's ability to regurgitate the procedures and principles taught in class. Creativity and trying new ways of caring for patients are not fostered or promoted to a great enough degree. It seems that this type of conformity is promoted in nursing as a cautionary measure to protect the patient. While it would be irresponsible not to supervise the care students give, this can be carried to extremes. Also, in many settings, the issue is the character of the nurse rather than her knowledge and skill. When the focus is on her skill, it is still on whether or not she performs in the acceptable, traditional way. Many skills are taught in a specific way because that is the way the instructor learned to do it from her instructor. Procedures are not necessarily based on original experimentation. While many procedures have been tested over time and are effective, many others are carried out, it seems, because "that is the way it has always been done." Rather than question or experiment, students are often expected merely to conform to the usual way of doing things. This does not foster the kind of critical thinking that is necessary for the nurse to develop sound judgment and carry out independent actions as a professional.

Conformity and tradition are expressed in other ways in nursing. There are many symbols and symbolic behaviors left over from the Victorian era that do not seem to serve any useful purpose today. For example, many nurses who wear uniforms are required to wear starched caps. In the past, a cap was worn for sanitary purposes. It was also a custom in the past that women covered their hair with large caps while working. Some even wore nightcaps. It held the hair in place and kept it out of the woman's way as she went about her work, as well as keeping it clean. As customs and styles changed, the caps worn by nurses changed as well. The caps that adorn nurses today could hardly be said to serve any of those purposes. What happened is that the cap became a symbol. It identified the wearer as a professional nurse who had graduated from a particular school of nursing. When a patient saw someone in a white cap, he knew it was a nurse. Even this function is outdated now as many other groups of health care workers have donned "the cap." For example, many practical nurses and nurses' aides wear caps. Regardless of who wears a cap, it serves no useful purpose. If anything, it's uncomfortable, it's old-fashioned, and it's in the way when you are caring for patients. Those stiff, uncomfortable little white things that used to be lovingly referred to as our "dignity" outlived their usefulness years ago. Unfortunately, many people still tie up the wearing of a cap with professionalism — a poor analogy at best. In many mental health, ambulatory care and public health settings, nurses have given up these vestiges of the past. If wearing a cap is how we define our dignity and professionalism, we are in sad shape.

Symbolic behavior in nursing as a means of bringing about conformity is exemplified in the retention of rituals and ceremonies. Commencement ceremonies are often replete with traditional rituals. This may range from having students carry miniature lighted lamps (similar to the one carried by Florence Nightingale) to parading them down an aisle or across a stage to receive flowers, school pins, miniature caps, a white nurse's bible, etc. These rituals and symbols, while grotesquely outmoded, are still retained by many. The "Angel of Mercy" myth is still being perpetuated by such symbolism. It should be remembered that angels are nice — but they aren't human. Nursing needs to come down to earth. As long as we remain dewy-eyed, overly sentimental women who cling to traditions and symbols from the past, we will do little to change the image and the role of the nurse.

There are many ways that nurses pressure one another to conform to traditional behaviors. In the work setting, regardless of the type, individual nurses frequently work closely together. They have specific expectations of each other in regard to their work. Each observes how the other functions and behaves. If one of the nurses makes more independent decisions, she may be viewed by her peers as a rebel. She may be seen as careless or noncaring because she does not mold her behavior to the expectations of others. Because she is different, she may be viewed as a challenge or a threat by her co-workers. They may not recognize or give credence to her competency and she may be ostracized by the others. Somehow she will be given the message that she is not conforming to the status quo. When she needs assistance from her co-workers, she may find help a long time in coming, if at all. Or assistance may be given grudgingly — never willingly. Her suggestions or ideas will be overlooked or shrugged off. She may find herself going to lunch alone — and after everyone else has gone. Negative comments may be dropped about her to others — just enough to place her ability in question. Sometimes the rebel nurse succumbs to the pressure from others and conforms to their expectations. Isolation and group pressure are too much to cope with. She may then become one of those who maintain the status quo. It is easier. I wonder how many young nurses started out as independent, enthusiastic, inquisitive individuals who eventually succumbed to traditional expectations and behaviors?

Health care needs are rapidly increasing. Along with this are greater demands for new and better services. Our profession, in its attempts to help meet these needs, is changing in many significant ways. New and expanded roles are developing; new positions are being designed; new functions are being identified; new ideas and plans are being formulated. New and different systems are being implemented to deliver services. Some nurses, instead of viewing these changes as a challenge, heatedly debate the outcome of such changes. It is more comfortable to maintain things as they are. These individuals have been so well indoctrinated into their present roles and typical ways of functioning that doing something different is a serious threat. In a variety of ways they work to sabotage progress. One way that works fairly well is to complain to one another about changes that are taking place. The new way of doing something is compared to the old way and a forecast is made that "it will never work." Then they actively set about to prove this. Their resistance to change, to accepting new responsibilities or new ways of functioning, quietly inhibits growth and progress. Instead of being flexible and exploring new and more effective ways of doing things, "hardening of the arteries" sets in. They simply continue to function in traditional ways and give no recognition to the changes around them. This kind of conformity is common in all areas of nursing.

Sometimes resistance to new roles and functions in nursing are expressed very openly. Some nurses are very vocal about their lack of support for new ideas. They may simply criticize the change by challenging its feasibility. Dozens of reasons are cited as to why "it won't work." If this does not discourage the instigator of the change, she is "put down." The authenticity, practicality, competence or motivation of the change-agent is scrutinized and found to be wanting. By discrediting the person promoting change, the whole idea of change is discredited. This is a common instance of nurses policing other nurses in order to promote conformity.

On a more positive note, we can take pride in those situations in which nurses have worked together closely to identify unmet health needs of people and have developed new and expanded roles to meet those needs. Interestingly, we have had important examples of nurses working together in very cohesive and, therefore, effective ways for a long time. Unfortunately, these situations have not been well publicized or appreciated. For example, one of the oldest and most daring health care services offered in this country is that provided by the Frontier Nursing Service. It was

112 founded in 1925 by a pioneer nurse midwife, Mary Breckinridge, to provide health services to the mountain people who live in the rural backwoods of eastern Kentucky. The main transportation used by the nurses until recently was horses. These nurses travel across creeks, over mountains and through backwoods to deliver needed care and service to these medically indigent mountain folk. In 1972, over 22,000 patients were cared for by a team of forty-one nurses, four physicians and a pharmacist [11]. The nurses functioning in this setting have to be able to care for people with complex health problems, and they also provide a great deal of support for one another. They work closely with the people of the Appalachian mountains as well. The people have formed district committees through which they provide invaluable advice and assistance to the nurses [12]. Unless this group of people worked together cohesively, they would not be effective in providing the kind of health services needed by this small but isolated population. Certainly it could be said that the way these nurses are functioning does not conform to the traditional role of the nurse.

There are other exciting examples of nurses expanding their roles in rural areas where the only health care being provided to the poor and disadvantaged is through specific nursing projects. In Alaska, for example, thirty-five public health nurses are using dog teams to deliver health care in remote villages [13]. There are other examples of nurses setting up small but vital projects and clinics that provide needed services to forgotten and isolated groups of people around the country. The fact that these efforts are being made should demonstrate that breaking out of traditional roles will only take place when nurses learn to respect each other's competence and then to work together.

Another well-organized policing mechanism within our profession is the nursing hierarchy, made up of various people who have differing levels of responsibility, expertise and authority. There is usually an organized nursing hierarchy in agencies that provide nursing service and in schools of nursing. The authority that the individual has within this system is generally commensurate with the responsibility identified at any one level. For example, in many hospital settings the head nurse has the responsibility for managing a patient care unit. She therefore has the authority for making certain decisions regarding the operation of the unit. The supervisor usually has responsibility for many units. She has greater and usually broader authority for making and carrying out decisions. This pattern continues throughout the organization up to the director of nursing, who has responsibility for guiding and directing the activities within the total department. In many instances, this structure can be used to police other nurses. In its most negative sense, it is an organizational structure that promotes compliance and conformity. While this type of organization has its positive aspects (it is more efficient), it is probably one of the greatest re-inforcers of traditional roles and functioning for nurses. The on-going complex and varied responsibilities of a nursing department are so great that it is only reasonable to expect that some form of organization needs to be established. In some agencies, innovative experiments regarding new organizational patterns are taking place. Hopefully, these organizational patterns will be more effective than the outdated traditional models still operating in most settings. In these situations, nurses are encouraged to try new things rather than to conform to set patterns. Nurses at all levels work together and share in the decision-making process. New ideas are encouraged and respected. It is even acceptable for individuals to make mistakes. In these settings, it is understood that many times people learn better by trying new things and seeing for themselves that they are not workable or effective. Through experimentation, however, they often discover much more effective ways for getting work accomplished. In the traditional hierarchical pattern, many practices serve as a policing mechanism for nurses. Often the focus of these patterns has more to do with indirect patient care and organizational efficiency than direct patient care. For example, there may be strict dress codes requiring nurses to wear white uniforms, white hose and caps. The nurse who does not follow the code may be admonished by her immediate supervisor. On the basis of her appearance, she may be evaluated as "not very professional." Her over-all performance may be rated lower because of her nonadherence to the dress code. While I believe it is reasonable to expect a nurse or any other employee to use good judgment and common sense about her attire while at work, I do not believe it is appropriate in this day and age to equate this with professionalism. If anything, perhaps dress codes should be reevaluated and revised in keeping with contemporary nursing practice. I have seen references to past work performance of individual nurses that focused primarily on the appearance of the nurse. The fact that the nurse wore her uniform "too short" was the major focus of the evaluation, rather than her clinical skills in caring for patients.

Supervision of one nurse by another nurse is also an example of reinforcement of conformity to traditional functioning. Instead of supporting the initiative of some nurses to experiment with new ways of doing things, many nurses in supervisory positions expect the nurse to function in prescribed ways. Nurses are then evaluated in terms of whether or not they function according to established criteria that may be outdated and, in some cases, restrictive to effective and professional nursing practice. Along with this, there are often established procedures or policies which are supposed to provide guidelines for the nurse in her practice. All too often, these have outlived their original purpose and usefulness. They become institutionalized, however, and are carried out faithfully simply because they "have always been done." They are restrictive and interfere with accepted contemporary "professional" practices. At times, a sharp nurse will question why the procedure is necessary. Sometimes, she may even go so far as to trace where and why it originated. (Occasionally, she will be fortunate enough to uncover this information.) She may learn that at one time a specific problem occurred and that a procedure was developed to correct the situation. The procedure, over time, became carved in stone. The fact that it is no longer appropriate and, in fact, may create unnecessary work for the nurse is not challenged. How many times in the course of a day do we do certain tasks because they are just standard operating procedure of the past? The wasted human energy could be put to better use. It means, however, that more nurses will need to examine this area carefully and begin to ask "Why do we do this?" more often.

Schools of nursing have an organized hierarchy with authority concentrated at the upper levels that often promotes compliance and conformity. Most organizations today establish committees to meet specific goals and objectives within the organization. A smaller group of people are better able to focus on specific issues, reach a group consensus and make recommendations. In schools of nursing, just as in other organizations, there are various kinds of committees. Some have only minor importance, while others are of such significance that decisions made within the committee may affect the direction of the entire program or school operation. The assignment of faculty to these committees can be a means for promoting conformity and tradition. Here is how it works: Those faculty members with the greatest tenure, status or recognized power may be assigned to the most important committees. For example, in some schools the curriculum committee makes recommendations and decisions that will affect the rest of the faculty and the student body. If the individuals assigned to this committee are not forward-thinking, progressive and in tune with the times, a rather static, traditional curriculum will be maintained. Thus, through a small but powerful group of people, the philosophy and educational approach to preparing practitioners will be controlled and directed. The method, style and content for individual courses taught by individual faculty will be expected to conform to the total curriculum design. The aggressive, dynamic faculty member who pushes to change the curriculum or to include new and different materials and methods of teaching may find herself at odds with the "old guard." Her suggestions are met with resistance and sometimes hostility. Her requests to change the course she is teaching may be held up in lengthy committee discussions with prolonged delays. There may be several results. A decision is delayed for so long that the school year ends, and there is not adequate time left to prepare for the change even if it were to be approved. Or she may be told it is not possible to change her course because it would affect the total curriculum. The outcome results in maintenance of the same outdated traditional curriculum. In essence, a small group of people are able to police the activities and operation of the larger group through control established within a recognized committee. The same thing may occur in relation to other committees which focus on other important objectives.

Most faculty members would attest to the fact that just about everyone is assigned to some kind of a committee. In some schools, the faculty have the option to choose which committees they would prefer to work on. In others, they are assigned to committees which may or may not reflect their interest or their ability. In either case, it is common practice to require that faculty serve. This may then become a basis for the faculty being promoted or advanced within the organization. Sometimes the same senior

116 faculty are given preference for working on the most important committees. Junior faculty will find themselves on minor, less important committees which do little to change or redirect the activities of the school. Therefore, committee assignment is one method for promoting conformity and tradition. This same structure, within a progressive and dynamic system, may be used in the opposite way. It will be viewed as a mechanism for working toward innovative changes in a democratic manner. The special interests and talents of the faculty will be used to a much greater degree. Differing ideas and changes are welcome. The result is that the faculty have a sense of cohesiveness and esprit de corps. And the curriculum is progressive and in tune with societal needs.

Nursing faculty, like other women, police their individual peers and exert pressure to conform to accepted modes of behavior. For example, on many faculties, association with students other than in the classroom or clinical areas is "frowned" upon. Also, the way in which the faculty member is expected to relate to and communicate with students is clearly established. In both areas, formality and distance are expected in order to maintain objectivity in relation to the student. The fact that each faculty member has a unique and distinct style of communicating and relating to others is not considered. The fact that the faculty member is a well-educated adult, capable of taking responsibility for her own actions, is not appropriately acknowledged. The individual faculty member who refuses to abide by these codes of behavior may find herself ostracized by her peers. Worse yet, she may be counseled by her department head or the dean. The fact that students respect her, enjoy her course and are highly motivated to learn may do little to enhance the situation. Most students would tell us that they have no desire to become "big buddies" with their teachers. They would, however, like to relate to them in more personal and human ways. The teacher who is cool, detached and unapproachable is often feared by students. This can and does interfere with the learning process. Since learning should be fun, it seems reasonable to expect that both the teacher and the learner should have the freedom to approach the educational process in less rigidly defined ways.

There are many other examples that could be cited to illustrate how the hierarchy in nursing, both in health care agencies and in schools, serves as a policing mechanism among nurses. While a great deal of time seems to be spent on policing the behavior and action of other nurses, all too often those individuals in the hierarchy do not police the health care system on behalf of the patients. Nursing educators spend much of their time policing students and other faculty instead of the educational system. As long as nurses continue to pressure one another to conform to outdated traditional molds, we will not only be forced to tolerate mediocrity in our profession but we will in essence be *promoting* mediocrity. Instead of policing one another, we need to develop systems of peer review. Peer review is the process by which registered nurses who are actively engaged in the practice of nursing assess the quality of nursing care in specific situations in keeping with established standards for nursing practice. The purposes of peer review are: to evaluate the quality and quantity of nursing care; to identify the strengths and weaknesses of nursing care; to present evidence to be used as a basis for recommending changes in policies or procedures to improve nursing care; to identify areas in practice patterns that indicate a need for increased knowledge. The process of peer review includes the appraisal of nursing care delivered by individual nurse practitioners as well as groups of nurses in a given setting [14]. It is a mechanism that promotes evaluation and accountability among professional nurses for the care they give to others. It is not a punitive process; the policing of nurses by other nurses to conform to outmoded traditional practices is. We must move as a profession from policing practices to peer review.

Competition
Competition abounds in the nursing profession just as it does in other female-dominated groups. Some competition is healthy and constructive. It challenges us to try new things, to be enthusiastic, to pursue new goals energetically. Other kinds of competition have a destructive force that prevents nurses from working together. Instead, we see nurses working against one another. A tremendous amount of time, energy and emotion gets tied up in the competitive struggles that go on between various nurses and nursing groups. The old adage "divide and conquer" comes to mind when thinking about the many ways that nurses compete with one another. Because we are divided in our thinking on many issues, our energy

118 seems to be tied up in showing each other how right we are on our particular stand. We work to discredit others who have the opposite viewpoint. In the meantime, the whole health care system is in disarray. Our profession has the potential to play a more significant role in reshaping the system, but as long as nurses are in disharmony with one another, feel isolated from each other and continue to perpetuate destructive competition, we will never fully utilize our potential for making necessary changes in health care.

There are a number of examples of competition among nurses within the profession. One of the most obvious, and the most controversial, are the questions that have raged in our profession for over two decades: the type and duration of nursing education. The first school of nursing in the United States was Bellevue Hospital School of Nursing, established in 1873. Up until 1962, approximately 80 percent of all nursing school graduates were from hospital diploma programs [15]. The remaining nurses were prepared in associate degree or baccalaureate programs. In 1964, the American Nurses' Association prepared a position paper regarding nursing education for the future. It proposed that all nursing preparatory programs eventually be located in institutions of higher education. It also recommended that the remaining hospital schools be phased out according to a specific, organized plan [16]. This marked the beginning of a furor that continues unabated. The dust may never settle over this issue! The opponents of the position paper argue that the hospital-based program prepares the best clinical practitioner. It is contended that these programs have a built-in emphasis on patient care and clinical experience. The proponents, on the other hand, argue that there are academic advantages within the regular educational institutions that are not available in hospital-based schools. For example, the nurse prepared in an institution of higher education has a broader educational base and has exposure to students in other fields. It is also pointed out that nursing is the only profession that does not prepare all its practitioners in institutions of higher education, one of the established standards for a profession [17].

As soon as the position paper was published, reaction was immediate and emotional on both sides of the issue. As emotions intensified, positions regarding the matter hardened. The battle was on — and still is. Charges and countercharges have been abundant over the past ten years. And everyone seems to be in on the act. Physicians, hospital administrators, nursing educators, practicing nurses and students — all have opinions on the best way to educate a nurse. Physicians and hospital administrators seem to prefer hospital-prepared nurses; nursing educators are divided; practicing nurses usually align themselves with the type of program they went through; students defend the type of program they affiliate with; the public — they are totally confused. It isn't enough that no one seems to agree on any of this, but the argument has kept nursing in a competitive, divided state for ten years. This divisiveness is perpetuated in an insidious manner at the functional level on an almost daily basis. Nurses who were prepared in one of the three different types of programs practice side by side in various settings, and comparisons are discussed among them. Innuendos and sometimes direct devaluation of an individual nurse's particular educational background are pointed out. The competition and struggle between nursing educators is carried on by the graduates in the work world. I talked to a young graduate not long ago who terminated her employment in one setting because she was made to feel inferior by her co-workers, who were all graduates of the other two types of educational programs. This is a sad commentary on our profession. I work with graduates from all three types of preparatory programs. My personal bias is that each has something unique to offer. There are outstanding practitioners from all programs — and there are poor practitioners from all programs as well. The question is not "who is best?" but rather "who can do what in the best way?" We are all nurses, and we must learn to work together. We must learn to respect the individual talents and competence of each practitioner — regardless of her background. Instead of setting up competitive, castelike structures in nursing, we should lay this issue to rest and start working together in more constructive ways.

While everyone has been battling over this controversial issue for the past decade, there has been a large reduction in the number of hospital schools with a resultant lowering of graduates from diploma programs. By 1972, the number of students graduating from diploma programs had declined from 80 percent to 41.7 percent. This represents about half of what it was in 1962. In

120 the meantime, the numbers of graduates from associate degree
programs have soared. By 1972, the percentage of associate degree
graduates had increased to 10 times the percentage in 1962 [18].
Many people are quick to credit the American Nurses' Association
position paper for this change in preparing nurses. It has been
pointed out, however, that trends toward restructuring educational
patterns in America started after World War II. To begin with, we
are moving toward a norm of 14 years of general education for our
nation. There has been a growing public trend to support and to
attain expectations for higher education. Institutions that offer a
general curriculum as well as vocational preparation are replacing
single-purpose or largely vocational institutions. The fact that
hospital schools are being replaced by collegiate institutions merely
illustrates the natural educational evolution within our culture.
Other problems related to financing and recruitment of faculty
and students have also contributed to the partial demise of hospital
schools of nursing [19]. The pains of change are often great.
Instead of expending energy on defensive competitiveness, nursing
educators should be working toward methods to facilitate articula-
tion between various aspects of the nursing education system. Basic
to this issue is the philosophy that education must be an open-
ended process and that every individual has the right to access to
enlarged opportunities for education [20].

There are other examples of competition within our profession.
It occurs in health care agencies as well as schools of nursing. I
have pointed out in previous chapters that there is a shortage of
nurses in all areas: in service agencies, in schools of nursing and in
leadership roles. It is rare to hear anyone say that they have an
adequate number of nurses regardless of the type of work setting.
Professional journals are filled with ads hoping to recruit staff
nurses, inservice education coordinators, faculty, directors and
assistant directors, public health nurses, deans, school nurses, etc.
The local newspaper provides a similar picture. Some larger institutions have professional nurses on their staff whose sole responsibility is to recruit nurses. Very appropriately, this individual's
title is "nurse recruiter." A great deal of money is spent on advertising using a variety of sometimes very creative methods for
recruitment. Because there is a shortage of nursing womanpower,
the institutions that employ nurses are placed in competition with

administrator in competition with her own colleagues. Frequently, each administrator who has responsibility for recruiting and hiring nurses works alone in her efforts to recruit the needed staff. The need may become so great and the competition so tough that these administrators sometimes make promises to prospective employees that later cannot be carried out. The result is a disillusioned and unhappy nurse who may jump back on the treadmill of job-hopping. Another problem that occurs is that the particular interest and expertise of the nurse may not be appropriately utilized because of inadequate staffing. For example, the prospective nurse may be interested in working with children. This has been her past experience, and she is skilled in this area. The administrator may be under pressure to hire more nurses for the coronary care unit, as it is understaffed. That is not what the nurse is interested in, nor does she have any experience in this area. The administrator may then hire the nurse and assign her to the coronary care unit with the idea that she will be transferred to her preferred area when more staff are hired. In many instances this does not work out, for obvious reasons. The nurse may leave or start looking for another job. In the meantime, across town (or even up the street) another administrator has similar problems. The two do not pool their resources or share ideas for coping with their mutual problem — inadequate staffing. Instead, they compete with one another. Sometimes the competition becomes so great that individuals may use extraordinary tactics to lure staff to their agencies. In terms of leadership it seems that the most important aspect of the recruiter's job is to find competent nurses to function in roles that they are suited for and interested in, and then to pay them an equitable salary. Instead of competing for such individuals, nursing administrators might be more successful if they pooled their ideas and resources and worked together. They could all benefit from this type of relationship and would have a greater opportunity for meeting their individual staffing needs. There are resourceful administrators who have done this with a great degree of success.

Schools of nursing are also in competition for attracting faculty. They compete with other schools as well as the various health care agencies. Similar problems occur as with other nursing administrators. The dean of the school is in competition with her colleagues to attract adequate numbers of qualified faculty. Often, she works alone in this area instead of working with other nursing administrators in her area. She may also develop tactics to recruit faculty, and she may make promises that cannot be fulfilled. Many times, in the struggle to hire the number of faculty needed, individuals are hired who lack the appropriate credentials and background experience for teaching. Both the faculty and the student body suffer the consequences.

Another area in which there is obvious competition is between the two professional organizations. The American Nurses' Association and the National League for Nursing have been competing for a long period. Both organizations have a long and proud history. The National League for Nursing was the first official organized group of nurses, established in 1894 under the name of the American Society of Superintendents of Training Schools for Nurses and made up entirely of educators. One of the main reasons it was organized was to establish and maintain badly needed universal standards for educating nurses. It was reorganized and given its present name in 1952. In 1896, Elizabeth Hampton Robb, who was a firm believer in the power of organized effort, founded the Associated Alumnae of the United States and Canada. Since practitioners of nursing at that time were not united and not included in the N.L.N., she set out to form an organization that would bring all nurses together to focus on their general needs and common welfare. In 1911, the name of the organization was officially changed to the American Nurses' Association [21]. Since their early beginning, both organizations have been dedicated to important goals that affect the education and practice of nurses and ultimately the health care of people.

A.N.A. membership consists only of registered nurses and is recognized as the official professional organization that represents all nurses. Membership in the N.L.N., on the other hand, is made up of nurses, agencies and consumers. Both groups are concerned about quality health care for the public. The N.L.N. has primarily focused on educational concerns such as accreditation, while the A.N.A. has focused on practice standards and general welfare of nurses as well as educational concerns. For many years, there have been debates concerning the pros and cons of having one organization for nurses that could speak for us with one united voice. Many nurses belong to both organizations. This confirms one of the arguments for combining the two organizations, as many individuals are investing time and energy in two directions and duplication in some areas, which wastes time, effort and talent. Heated debates have continued, however, with no realistic resolution of the argument.

One of the most vexing issues between the two organizations involves the issue of accreditation of basic and graduate nursing education programs. The purpose of accreditation is to foster excellence through specific standards, assess educational effectiveness, ensure quality, encourage institutional improvement through self-study and planning and to protect against encroachment. Long ago it was decided that accreditation for nursing education should be the joint function of the schools, nurses and the public. For this reason, then, the accreditation process was placed under the jurisdiction of the National League for Nursing. It was felt at the time that if the American Nurses' Association assumed this responsibility, accreditation would become a function of nurses alone [22]. The N.L.N. has carried out this responsibility since that time, and improvements have been made in all types of nursing education programs. In the meantime, many nurses have been embroiled in the matter of who should be responsible for this function.

The issue came to a head in 1974 at the A.N.A. convention, when the House of Delegates passed a resolution which directed the A.N.A. Board of Directors to "move with all deliberate speed to establish a system of accreditation of continuing education programs in nursing and [for the A.N.A. to] move just as expeditiously to examine the feasibility of accreditation of basic and graduate education [23]. The reasoning behind this resolution was the strong feeling by the delegates that one of the distinguishing characteristics of a profession is autonomy and self-regulation in matters that affect its practice and education. It was further pointed out that the responsibility for regulating nursing education presently rests with an organization (the N.L.N.) separate and apart from the professional society. On the other hand, it was felt that the A.N.A., as the recognized professional nursing society, was willing and able to assume this function on behalf of the profession. Since that action was taken, there have been more heated debates between both organizations. I have received many position papers from the National League for Nursing stating their position on the issue and criticizing the action taken by the delegates. I have read many position statements by the A.N.A. concerning the issue in its official publication *The American Nurse.*

To date the issue has not been resolved, and it seems that both groups have valid points for their particular stand. While many individual nurses are still strongly debating this question, interested groups have finally started holding conferences to attempt to compromise and resolve the issue at last. Early this year, representatives of agencies that are interested in the accreditation of nursing programs met to prepare a formal proposal for a study regarding the feasibility of the American Nurses' Association assuming responsibility for the accreditation of basic and graduate nursing education. Among the groups were the National League for Nursing, the American Association of Colleges of Nursing, the American Nurses' Association, American Association of Nurse Anesthetists, a state board of nursing representatives and others. If this group, through their action, reinstitutes the use of interorganizational means of collaboration to resolve this controversial issue in nursing, it would serve as an excellent example of unity. Instead of perpetuating competition and devisiveness, this action could serve to bring us together to speak with one voice instead of many "tongues" [24]. Succinctly stated by Margretta Styles, "We shall be *vulnerable* or *invincible* depending upon our unity, our public visibility, our self image, our reality orientation, our activisim, our product development and salesmanship and our accountability" [25].

On Success

Another characteristic that distinguishes nurses' relationships with one another is their motivation to avoid success. Just as with other women, many nurses seem to fear success in other than traditional roles. (This notion will be dealt with more fully in a later chapter.) While successful nurses still seem to be the exception rather than the rule, we do have examples of nurses who have been defined as successful by some. These women could be termed the Queen Bees in nursing.

The Queen Bee syndrome developed by some nurses is diagnosed by characteristic symptoms. To begin with they are different from many other nurses. They are not ordinary in the area of motivation and achievement. They are talented individuals who have excelled in their chosen area of interest. This could be in a specific practice area, in the area of education or research or in some aspect of administration or management. Their contributions in any one of these areas are recognized as significant. They are usually respected for their expertise and knowledge and are viewed by others in the nursing community as successful. They also view themselves as successful. They think of themselves as different from other nurses and do not want to associate closely with their own group. Like other Queen Bees they want to identify up, not down, and therefore they identify with others outside of nursing. Very often, these others are men. One of the reasons they may want to identify with men who are outside of nursing is because part of their success could be attributed to men in the system where they are located. They then maintain an allegiance to these men and to the system. Queen Bees in nursing are usually found to hold the higher paying, more prestigious positions (in nursing, that is). They do not necessarily hold positions that are as well-paying and prestigious as men have in the same system. In comparison to their nursing colleagues, however, they may have a decided advantage. Since the Queen Bees enjoy a privileged position (especially for a nurse), they are not necessarily concerned about making changes in the system they are in. They enjoy their special position and work very hard to maintain it. Other nurses are viewed as "competition." Since they worked very hard to attain their position and status, they do not want other nurses to obtain the same level without a great deal of effort, and they give little assistance or encouragement to younger nurses. They are, in fact, the enemy. They are not sensitive to the problems of their own colleagues and do not relate to them in other than superficial and competitive ways. They see themselves as individualists who work primarily alone or with men in the system. Much of what they do is for personal gratification and recognition. They have their own set of strategies for meeting these goals. Working in groups with other nurses is not only difficult but, at times, impossible. They do not see the problems in nursing as a total group problem or their problem. Rather, they see the many problems of nursing as a problem of individual nurses. Their attitude is "I've gotten where I am by myself. Their problems are their own. If they really wanted to do something about their situation, they would." Because of their attitude, their isolation from other nurses and their lack of

126 relatedness to nurses and nursing, they will do little to help their peers. Their energy will be invested in maintaining things as they are. They will continue to align themselves with those who help to maintain their special position and status. They will work aggressively to divert or discredit other talented nurses who could pose a threat to their enviable position.

It is very frustrating to work with a Queen Bee. To begin with, if she is in a position of authority, she demands allegiance from others to her rather than to an idea, a program or the profession. If she has special skills, she will not teach other nurses those skills; she keeps them to herself. If she is in a practice setting working with a patient who has special needs that she cannot meet, she will not refer the patient to a nursing colleague; she will find someone else after she finally decides that she herself cannot do it. Some Queen Bees will work with groups of nurses, but only on certain levels. They will either have to be the "star attraction" who receives special treatment and recognition, or they will have to "run the show." The decision to get involved with other nurses is made on the basis of how it will benefit the Queen Bee — not how others might benefit.

Somewhere in life, I was taught that the most productive competition is that which one engages in with one's self. It seems to me that well-adjusted, mature individuals are those who know what their own potentials and limitations are and how best to utilize both to accomplish what it is they want to do in life. That means that the individual competes with himself to meet his goals — whatever they are. To view others continually as a threat or a source of personal competition indicates that the individual's self-concept and sense of self-esteem are not very strong or positive. I have met and worked with some extraordinary women in my life. They were positive role models for me because their greatness came not from competing with other women in destructive and devisive ways but rather was a result of their special talents and abilities, which they shared with others. They were aggressive, competent women who were able to teach and to share with others in an honest and fair way. They respected themselves and they respected others. I wanted to be like them because they were strong women. Because they valued themselves as women, they were able to value me. And I learned a great deal from them.

Women everywhere are beginning to think about themselves — and other women. They are beginning to explore new ways of communicating and relating to one another. They are beginning to see that other women have the same problems and concerns that they themselves have. As more women get together to share ideas, concerns, hang-ups, frustrations, etc., they will begin to realize the political nature of their complaints. In the past, these things were discussed as trivial or strictly personal. Women, including nurses, who have had an opportunity to share their feelings with other women on a deeper, noncompetitive level have benefited from the tender, compassionate understanding and support they have received. This has enabled many to focus more critically on their role as a woman and to initiate political strategies that will bring about the kind of social changes that will promote equality for women in all areas.

We as nurses have enviable opportunities to cross the barriers of age, economics, experience, race and culture to make deep and personal connections with other women — whether they be friends, co-workers, colleagues or patients.

References

1. Steinem, Gloria. Sisterhood. *Ms.,* Preview Issue, Spring, 1972, p. 48.
2. Chesler, Phyllis. Are We a Threat to Each Other? *Ms.,* Vol. I, No. 4, October 1972, p. 89.
3. Steinem, Gloria, op. cit., p. 49.
4. Bardwick, Judith M., and Douvan, Elizabeth. Ambivalence — the Socialization of Women. In *Woman in Sexist Society: Studies in Power and Powerlessness,* Gornick, Vivian, and Moran, Barbara (Eds.). New York: Basic Books, 1971, p. 231.
5. Kundsin, Ruth. To Autonomous Women: An Introduction. In *Women and Success: The Anatomy of Achievement,* Kundsin, Ruth (Ed.). New York: William Morrow, 1974, p. 11.
6. Epstein, Cynthia Fuchs. Bringing Women In: Rewards, Punishments and the Structure of Achievement. In *Women and Success: The Anatomy of Achievement,* Kundsin, Ruth (Ed.). New York: William Morrow, 1974, p. 13.
7. Kundsin, Ruth, op. cit., p. 12.
8. Staines, Graham, Tavris, Carol, and Jayaratne, Toby Epstein. The Queen Bee Syndrome. *Psychology Today,* Vol. 7, No. 8, January 1974, p. 55.
9. Ibid., pp. 57–60.
10. Massachusetts Nurses Battle a Relaxed License Law. *American Journal of Nursing,* Vol. 73, No. 6, June 1973, pp. 961, 963.

128 11. Kushner, Trucia. The Nursing Profession — Condition: Critical. *Ms.*, Vol. II, No. 2, August 1973, p. 100.
12. Tirpak, Helen. The Frontier Nursing Service — Fifty Years in the Mountains. *Nursing Outlook,* Vol. 23, No. 5, May 1975, p. 309.
13. Ibid., p. 100.
14. Peer Review Guidelines Proposed. *The American Nurse,* Vol. 5, No. 7, July 1973, pp. 1, 5.
15. *Facts About Nursing 72—73.* Kansas City, Mo: American Nurses' Association, 1974.
16. Lysaught, Jerome. *An Abstract for Action.* New York: McGraw-Hill, 1970, pp. 6, 101—102.
17. Ibid., pp. 6, 103, 104.
18. American Nurses' Association, op. cit., pp. 70—71.
19. Lysaught, Jerome, op. cit., pp. 104—105.
20. Ibid., p. 116.
21. Christy, Teresa. Nurses in American History, The Fateful Decade, 1890—1900. *American Journal of Nursing,* Vol. 75, No. 7, July 1975, p. 1164.
22. Pitchford, Mary. ANA Holds First Accreditation Conference. *The American Nurse,* Vol. 7, No. 1, January 1975, pp. 1, 7—8.
23. Ibid., p. 1.
24. Ibid., pp. 7—8.
25. Ibid., p. 7.

5 The Art of Saying No

Marlene Grissum

I regard people who say No as more real than people who don't — and I like real people [1].

Henry Close

The ability to say no is an art in the sense that art is a human skill —
just as to nurse is an art — a skill that can be learned, then nurtured
and nourished until it grows.

Women are becoming aware of the barriers in society that prevent them from developing their full potential, one of those barriers
being the weak sense of self-esteem that makes them unable to say
no. Knowing how and when to say no is probably one of the most
difficult arts/skills we humans must learn. (Of course, there is the
period of "the terrible two's" when no seems to be the only word
in our vocabulary; this will be discussed later in the chapter.)
This chapter deals mainly with how, why and when it is essential
and appropriate for nurses to say no; it attempts to show that this
skill is indeed related to our sense of self-worth, others' perceptions
of our worth and our concept of ourselves as nurses; and it also
shows that an inability to say no leaves us powerless, without
autonomy and with a sense of worthlessness, particularly in regard
to our profession.

All of us, women and men, have difficulty in saying no to certain people, but it is doubly difficult for women. Therefore, it is doubly important that we learn how to, when to and for what reasons. In explaining the how, why and when of saying no, we will also be exploring those facets of self-worth (or lack of it) that provide us with the strength to deal with the emotional stress of saying no. Learning to say no is not an isolated learning experience. It is an integral part of human growth and development that begins in early childhood when the young child first begins to affirm her separateness — usually around the age of two years. As she begins to realize that she is separate — a person unto herself — she gradually manifests her independence, particularly by saying no. The business of asserting independence is so strong in some children that it seems they never say anything else but no. They rarely agree with any plan suggested to them — even if they want to do whatever it is. This reaches such unreasonable proportions at times that the whole year has been labeled "the terrible two's" by parents and other child-rearing authorities. Having guided four daughters through the terrible two's, I can say that a more apt label could not have been found. To watch one small human begin the long, hard struggle to define her sense of self is both exasperating and joyous. Certainly, at times, it must be frightening to the child. After all, to be independent, one must give up the security of being dependent. Women therefore should recognize that we still have difficulty in asserting independence because we have been socialized to be dependent. "I don't need to say No to people. If I ever get into difficulty, somebody will rescue me. As long as I don't say No, I maintain my dependent ties with other people, and they are responsible for me" [1].

The idea of children asserting their independence is frightening and threatening to many parents, and some even take this to mean that the child is saying they are not good parents. In order to decrease their own sense of unworthiness, parents begin to smother the child's growing sense of independence by enforcing stricter rules and demanding more rigid obedience. Sometimes they are so threatened and frightened by the child's behavior (which they perceive as losing control over the child) that they withdraw their love and support. Either way, the child may very well interpret

the parents' behavior as indicating that independence is bad — and
not a good thing for them to learn. In the process, they grow up
believing that to say no means they will no longer be nice people
and that they will not be liked or loved. "Nice people don't say
No to other people. Since I am a nice person I can never say No
to anyone. It would ruin my image of myself, and I would be
terribly embarrassed" [1]. When one adds this concept to those
already discussed in the chapter on the socialization of women, it
is not difficult to understand why women have problems in dealing
with the art of saying no. But what most women have really never
thought about is that "if we can't say No we can't really say Yes
either" [1]. Both answers grow out of our sense of being a real
person — of affirming ourselves and controlling our own lives. "To
be *real,* in a psychological sense, means to be integrated — integrated
in thought, feeling and bodily behavior" [2]. To paraphrase Brandon,
woman is not a disembodied intellect, and she is not merely a mind
that happens to inhabit a body. Woman is an organism — a living
entity — who is conscious; which is to say, she is a person [2]. It
is only when we can incorporate this thought into our inner self
that we can begin to see that we can say no without losing more
than we gain.

All persons have some degree of self-worth — it varies among
individuals and within individuals but it is a part of every person.
Woman's sense of self-worth has been a sadly neglected part of our
socialization process. And our sense of unworthiness leads us to
say yes many times. "Only people who are really worth something
have the right to say No. I am not worthy of that. My wishes are
not that important. My sense of worth comes only from serving
other people" [1]. It is our feelings of unworthiness that lead
women to say "I'm only a housewife" or "I'm just a woman" or
"Yes, if *you* think I can" or "My opinion is not worth much." Our
sense of unworthiness allows us to be blackmailed into always saying
yes. Because women are socialized to be givers, because motherhood is still our ultimate goal, because our society declares
that *good mothers* have the capacity for unlimited giving, women
grow up believing they have no right to say no. The woman's image
of herself as an unworthy person makes it difficult to say no, and
the male-dominated (and to a lesser degree, child-dominated)
society capitalizes on that difficulty every day. For example:

The Art of Saying No

134 Women are perceived by both men and women as being compassionate, tender and nurturant. Society often takes advantage of people with these qualities. This is such a widespread phenomenon that businesses play upon it, especially through advertising; charitable organizations depend upon it for both funds and volunteers; and our loved ones rely upon it to get them out of tight squeezes. Our inability to say no, even when we would like to, stems from the fact that we are not self-actualized — we have less sense of self-esteem, we feel we are worth less than the really important people in the world, i.e., men. So, instead of asserting ourselves by saying no when asked to volunteer for some task that men would be paid to do — we do it for nothing and feel even less worthy. If, for some reason, we cannot possibly squeeze one more thankless job into our daily lives, we feel so guilty that we frequently give money in a vain attempt to assuage our guilt for having said no. Strange as it may seem to most women, your child will not fail the third grade if you refuse to be room mother! (And why don't they have room fathers?) The election of the political candidate of your choice will be neither won nor lost by his/her paying you a fair wage for the hard labor of a campaign. "In 1965 an economist estimated the monetary worth of volunteer work, at 14.2 billion dollars" [3].

Why is it so difficult for women to say no when they see their sisters go off to some volunteer job or they are asked to participate in some fund-raising drive? According to Gold, it is because they feel a "powerful social disapproval coupled with their own psychological conditioning of self-negation and ambivalent self-realization" [3]. In other words, they have such a lack of self-esteem and are so confused about their *real* selves that they cannot bear social disapproval, so they conform. Margaret Adams has defined this as "the compassion trap" [4]. She asserts: "It is one of the strongest forces in today's world that subverts and distorts both the individual identities and the social roles of women . . . It leads to an extremity of confused thinking as well as a great deal of frustrated and basically ineffectual activity" [4]. The idea that women's primary function is to be tender, compassionate, protecting and nurturing inhibits them from saying no to almost all demands, even those that are frequently unreasonable and almost always exploitive. Learning how to say no may be the first step in springing the catch on the compassion trap, thereby freeing us to live our lives as truly *free*

right to a self that is actualized (i.e., more integrated, more fully
human). As the self develops, a realization that *I own myself*
begins to grow within us. Without this feeling, we will remain self-
alienated, self-impoverished, with a sense of inner emptiness — a
"disowned self" [2]. With the realization that *I own myself* comes
the realization that *I do not own or owe anyone else.* If I neither
own nor owe anyone else, I can withstand their demands because
I am in charge of my own life and I am responsible for myself. I
have learned how to say no.

Saying no to those we love can be difficult at times. There are
so many other feelings woven into the warp and woof of love —
such as responsibility, compassion, guilt, respect and gratitude —
that it is sometimes necessary to pause and investigate why we are
saying yes or no. Perhaps all people, but particularly women, should
ask themselves, "Will my saying yes enrich my life, make my real
self more integrated, and will my saying yes do the same for the
person or persons making the demand?" In other words, will we
both gain, or will I become more of a *disowned self* and the others
weaker people because I have agreed to their demands? Whether
the loved one asking is your child who has attained adulthood but
still wants your financial support, or your husband who still expects
you to be his unpaid maid, or your friend who expects you to have
no other friends, the answer must still be based on the growth that
will occur to your self and the asker's self. As women learn to *own*
themselves, the answers will tend to be resounding no's. Women
will become positive forces in society to the extent that they come
to perceive themselves as having an identity and personal integrity
that has as strong a claim as any other individual or group for being
preserved intact [4].

I have been dealing with the concept of saying no as it relates
to women in general. By so doing, I have implied that women are
married, have children, stay at home and give away their time. We
all know, however, that that implication is not real. In reality,
over 40 percent [5] of the work force in the United States are
women. Are they in any better position to say no than their sisters
who stay at home? The answer seems to be that they are not —
women still have difficulty in asserting themselves. They may have
exchanged situations as to what kinds of demands are put to them,

but the demands are still there. "Even women who pursue a career or profession, rather than merely holding a meaningless job, assume the responsibility for two major, demanding roles" [6]. The characteristics that supposedly make women successful in the home and tend to pressure them into always saying yes — their compassion, their ability to sustain and support others, their willingness to give — tend to be their undoing in the world of work. In many instances, even the woman's work is for giving purposes. For example, her income is likely to be viewed by others as supplemental, a help but not absolutely essential to the family welfare. Most likely it will be used to contribute to family vacations, college fees or some luxury for the home. Whether her job is demeaning or exciting, needed for essentials or used for luxuries, she gives. There are no no's in most women's lives except those they hear from significant others. For the woman to deny others is to deny herself, because she has no real Self — she has been taught to give it all away. Hence, she has no right to say no because she has nothing to say no with — all of *her* belongs to others; however, she has no right to say yes either, because she cannot give away what she does not own. Someone else will then have to say yes for her, whether that someone is society who says it is acceptable for women to *give* their time and talents but unacceptable to sell them for a good salary, or whether it is a husband who says it is acceptable for a wife to work as long as she only *supplements* income and does not neglect her "real" duties as wife and mother.

Once the woman does go to work, how does her inability to say no influence her ability to perform her job? All of us who work — men and women — know that in most instances there are at least a few people to whom we cannot say no if we want to continue to work at that particular job. But again, women allow themselves to be put in double jeopardy. Because we have very little sense of self-worth, we are willing to take jobs at less pay — jobs that are demeaning, boring, demoralizing and exploitive. Frequently, we rationalize this by saying, "Oh well, I don't have to do it for long. As soon as my children are educated I'll quit." Because we are not highly motivated, do not know what is normal or desirable in the work field, do not have a high regard for our self and have little or no idea what we are worth in terms of dollars, we sell ourselves short both as a person and a potential source of income for ourselves

and our family. In short, we cannot say no to an employer's offer **137**
to work for less money than he would have to pay a man. The
first time I ever refused to work for the salary offered, my potential
employer was amazed. It was the first time he had *ever* heard a
woman say, "No, I'd rather go hungry than to sell my skills for
that amount of money!" When he realized that not only was I
insulted by his offer, but I meant what I said, he began serious
negotiations with me regarding the job. Several times since then,
I have either refused jobs or quit jobs over money. Each time people
around me are always somewhat skeptical regarding my reasons.

It never occurs to many people that a nurse — a person *dedicated*
to serving humankind — could possibly be interested in money —
let alone be so selfish as to put her own interests above her profession! It is just as amazing, however, that they have never realized
that a nurse can perform her duties just as well, if not better, for
a fair salary as for a low one. The idea that nurses give their skills
and talents because they are dedicated to caring for the ill and the
infirm is left over from the dark ages when religious orders were
founded for that purpose. It is a myth that is continued in our
society because it is to men's advantage to perpetuate it and women
(nurses) are too weak to say no. Nurses, probably more than any
other work group, are extremely vulnerable to all the nuances of
the compassion trap. It leads nurses to misplace a great deal of
vital energy, which in turn leads them to being self defeating. It
also results in society's being deprived of their significant contributions to the health care of this country. Their inability to say
no because they are not *self-owned* individuals and the fact that
they are caught in the compassion trap increase their frustration
to the point that they drop out of the profession. In this book,
statistics are cited several times on why nurses change jobs, leave
the field and generally disappear from the work force. Of course,
there is no single answer to such a complex question, but it does
seem that salary may be one of the answers. In many instances,
they may not have the courage — the sense of self — it takes to
say no in so many words, but they do say it in a more subtle form
when they simply refuse to work. They are, in a sense, saying no
to the whole relationship rather than to only one aspect of it.

The issue of salaries is not the only significant reason why nurses
say no; I use it merely as an example of one of the times nurses

138 can begin to say no in order to learn how, when and why no is an essential word for us to learn to use. Actually, money is probably the least important aspect of the relationship between nurses and the health care industry. But it does show that the monetary worth people place on a woman's work is an indication of the worth they place her personal self. Much more important, it is a reflection of our sense of personal worth when we sell our education and skills for less than their true value. This sense of personal worth — this sense of caring for self — is evidenced in a self-actualized person and allows that person to say no to one aspect of a relationship without saying no to the *whole*. A self-actualized nurse will not withdraw from her chosen profession. Instead, like the ethical person that James and Jongeward describe, she will "establish a practical, workable, concerned and enhancing relationship with [her] total environment" [7]. The problems will still be there and she will not discount their significance, but she will be able to work with others to solve them. Because she is a self-actualized person, however, she will be able to say no — in fact, it will be essential that she do this. In the process, decisions will have to be made by her as to when, where, how, why and to whom the answer no is appropriate. Ethics are an inherent part of every person, and certainly they are a part of every nurse. Just as with all situations that call for ethical consideration, a decision to say no must be based on ethics as well. "A decision is ethical if it enhances self-respect, develops personal integrity and integrity in relationships, dissolves unreal barriers between people, builds a core of genuine confidence in self and others, and facilitates the actualizing of human potentials without bringing harm to others" [7]. That may seem like a difficult task for nurses when it comes to making the decision to say no. It is not impossible, however, and most worthwhile endeavors are achieved only with some effort.

Achieving autonomy is the ultimate goal of a mature person. In order for nursing to become a mature profession, it too must have autonomy as its ultimate goal. In achieving autonomy and becoming self-actualized, we will learn to say no. Needless to say, it will cost us effort and energy, as well as the approval and support of some individuals and some groups. In reaching our goal, we will use every bit of stamina, integrity, strength and perseverance we have; but the end result will be a group that has the freedom to choose from a full spectrum of behaviors and feelings, and with our freedom of choice will come the ability to accept responsibility for that choice. Unless people make decisions such as these, their power remains undirected, unclear and unstable. "A person must do more, however, than make a decision. He must act on his decision or it is meaningless. Only when his inner ethics and outward behavior match and he is congruent is he a whole person. A spontaneous person is free 'to do his own thing' but not at the expense of others through exploitation and/or indifference" [7]. When one considers how many people are exploited in this world, one wonders if there really are any persons who are free, spontaneous, autonomous people. That thought does not negate the fact that we all *could be* if we were willing to begin the process by knowing our self.

The autonomous person does not need to exploit others in order to achieve the sense of worth necessary to "make it" with society as a whole or with himself. Neither does the person have to be the self-effacing, self-sacrificing and self-seeking person that many women are. Often, by never having the courage to say no, we manipulate others by making them feel obligated to us. This is so prevalent in nursing it is almost endemic to any relationship where nurses are involved. One wonders just how many nurses there are who build their whole practice (and their own little queendom) on the premise that "if I take care of them (other health care professionals) and do favors for them, I can expect them to reciprocate and take care of me." I have observed this many times, particularly in hospital settings, where nurses build this manipulative relationship with doctors in the hope that the doctors will then "protect" them from the administration, including nursing administration. Usually it is one nurse who does this, and more than likely she will manage to develop the relationship with only one or two physicians. She makes sure their orders are carried out first and their patients are taken better care of — their wishes are her commands. She would not dream of saying no to them, even to the extent that she will give preferential care to their patients and neglect others. She is self effacing and self sacrificing to the point of doing nothing except what she perceives is pleasing to them. In establishing such a relationship, she hopes, consciously or unconsciously, that she can become totally dependent upon them. They will fight her battles; she will have no need ever to develop the sense of Self needed to say no — they will do it for her. All she has to do is tell them whatever demands someone else makes on her, and they will go to battle for her. By so doing, though, she loses her own chances for self actualization and increases other nurses' difficulties in establishing their own autonomous identity.

As we learn more direct ways of establishing relationships with other health care professionals, we can give up the manipulation of never saying no. Nurses' becoming autonomous may increase anxiety in some instances, but this is one area where physicians should be pleased with our liberation because they cannot enjoy being manipulated. Nor should they enjoy being in a pseudo-respectful relationship in which "respect" is actually built on the manipulative action and self sacrifice of others. "The autonomous person sacrifices only when he is sacrificing a lesser value for a greater value according to his own value system" [7]. Nurses need to become aware of the idea that they do not need any *one* person to give them approval and a sense of identity. Certainly, all humans need love and approval from others; but no *one* person can ever give us all the aspects of love and approval we need as persons, just as no one group of persons such as physicians can give all that is needed to another group such as nurses. Collectively and individually, we must establish a sense of identity within ourselves. Ultimately, love, approval and our own identity must come from within; however, nurses, like other women, need to learn the joy and sense of cohesiveness that can be achieved through support of each other. Generation after generation of women have been socialized to distrust other women as well as not to depend upon other women for approval and support. Nowhere is this easier to observe than in the field of nursing. For instance, an individual nurse is more likely to seek out the powerful support of her "favorite doctor" to lend credence to her demands than she is to seek it from the nursing organization of her health care agency. Nurses are almost as likely to seek validity for their practice by joining professional associations that are an "arm" of a medical specialty as they are to be certified through their own professional association.

We must know, love and approve of our own Self before we can gain these from others. A part of our being able to do this lies within our ability to say no, especially to those situations that will detract from our capacity to know ourselves. Just as we need to know that there are others who will continue to love and support us if one person threatens to withdraw his love, so we need to know others will support us if a group threatens to withdraw its approval and support. Nurses need to develop this knowledge of support within their own group. We can no longer afford to rely on others to support and protect us, as we have in the past. An autonomous person is a self-sufficient one, to the degree that self-sufficiency is possible. An autonomous profession must also be as self-sufficient as possible. If nurses, as a group and as individuals, truly wish to become autonomous, we must be responsible for our own decisions and the behavior that results from those decisions. We can no longer rely on hospitals to protect us from malpractice (a myth anyway), doctors to tell us how to perform nursing care or other personnel to do our work for us, just as we can no longer depend on medical specialties to give validity to our areas of expertise. By continuing any of these practices, we detract from ourselves as autonomous individuals and from our profession as an autonomous profession.

In order to accomplish a sense of cohesiveness and to lend support to others in our group, we must also learn to say no to ourselves. Next to saying no to others we love, saying no to ourselves (whom we also love) is most difficult. In essence, we must learn to control our impulses. We grow up learning how to control our harmful impulses; if we did not, we would become a menace to ourselves and to society. However, there are many impulses that *seem* perfectly harmless which nurses must learn to control, for instance, the impulse to ask for help outside our profession to solve our internal problems. Our first impulse may be to go to the administrator of the hospital, over the head of the nursing director, to solve a problem. It does not matter that up to this time the director has been totally ineffectual in solving our dilemmas. Perhaps it is because we have not presented a cohesive, supportive front for her to use in order to deal with the administration. If, in fact, she *is*

142 ineffectual and self effacing, perhaps it would be more effective if we exerted pressure by cohesiveness and let her know we expected her to behave as though she supports us. In other words, we need to say no to ourselves when we find ourselves depending on powerful men in the organization to fight our battles.

Another example of when we need to resist our impulses and say no to ourselves is when we are attacked by others in the health care field. Since most nurses are women and women tend not to fight back, we need to resist the impulse to give up — to run away — at the first sign of displeasure; and displeasure will be exhibited by physicians, administrators and other influential men in the health care industry when nurses start to become autonomous. When nurses start to assert themselves and take a stand for nursing, we will be attacked, not physically, but verbally at least. Verbal abuse is not easy to withstand either. We must be prepared for it, whether we are talking about individuals, health care agencies or the profession of nursing; we need to band together and support each other in the fight to raise nursing from its second-class status into the center of the health care industry. In order to do this, we will need to be able to resist the temptation of running away or selling out. Because we have been taught to be dependent both as nurses and as women, the effort to attain independence is a double one. First we must fight our own desire to remain dependent, and second, we must fight men's desire to keep us dependent. In order to do the fighting, we will have to say no to all the dependent behaviors we have.

In many instances it is much easier to remain dependent, or so it seems at times. For instance, it seems much easier to deal with just the medical problem of the patient as identified by the physician than to assess the whole patient in terms of what kind of nursing care that individual patient needs. The dependent nursing functions — medical orders — are so much easier to plan than the independent nursing functions — nursing orders — that our impulse may be to perform only those functions that the doctor has ordered. Say no to that impulse! In saying no to ourselves, we say no to the system that keeps us in the past. An autonomous person is aware of what is going on *now* [7]. We will never be an autonomous profession until the individuals within our profession become aware of the need to use our own knowledge base to make our own decisions concerning the kind of nursing care the patient needs. There was perhaps a time when nursing had no base of scientific knowledge to build upon or use in making well-thought-out decisions, but *now* that is no longer true. Not that we cannot use knowledge from other disciplines or that we are to ignore those dependent functions necessary to caring for patients. To do either is, again, letting our impulses rule our lives. But to rely totally on others' knowledge is to remain in the static, dependent state of the past. Autonomous persons and professions cannot and will not allow that to happen.

Another example of resisting the impulse to remain dependent is when nursing care plans are in opposition to medical care plans for a patient. If the patient-teaching is only half finished when the physician decides to discharge the patient, resist the impulse to say nothing, and say no instead! As people in our society become better educated in general, they have the capability to become better educated about their own state of health and how to maintain it. As we nurses become better educated, we have the capability (as well as the responsibility) to teach patients; however, we rarely do a really good job here because we are too dependent. We seldom discuss our plan of care for the patient with the physician and even more seldom with the patient. As a result, the patient is often discharged without our being informed beforehand. If nurses were able to resist their impulses to remain dependent, they could assert themselves enough to say no when physicians discharge patients at the completion of the medical care regimen without further instruction about after-care. Frequently, this results in patients being readmitted to the hospital several times for the same problem because they originally had gone home without adequate preparation for their own care. As hospitals become more and more acute-care-oriented, this will become an ever-increasing problem, and it will remain with us until we nurses resist the temptation to respond to our impulses. We must say no to such impulses.

Accepting "No" without Explanation

In learning to say no, we must learn to accept no from others. This seems as though it would be easy for most women; however, we are not used to hearing no as a self-actualized person, only as a

144 dependent, passive one. In our passive, dependent past we were often told no in a variety of ways for a variety of reasons, and many of us learned how to take a no and manipulate it into a yes as we became socialized to being a woman. As self-actualized, autonomous persons, we will reject manipulative behavior as unacceptable to our self-esteem. Not only will we need to resist the impulse to revert to manipulation, we must "remind ourselves that we don't own other people, and they do not owe us their favors or explanations. We are separate and independent" [1].

In our newly found sense of independence, being able to resist the temptation to *demand* an explanation for the no from others will be the true test of our autonomy. Now this may appear at first glance to be a paradox as well as a dilemma. It will seem at times that the two choices are equally negative. We can resist the impulse to demand an explanation, remain silent and thereby give the other person an opportunity to believe we are still a passive, dependent person, or we can speak out, demand the explanation and give in to our impulse to manipulate. Either avenue of escape is unacceptable to an autonomous person. One of the steps in learning to say no is making a deliberate commitment and following it through to the end, accepting all its consequences, and our ability to accept others' right to say no without an explanation is part of that commitment. I am not implying that there can be no communication between the two parties — there is no reason why the person who said no cannot give an adequate explanation for having done so, nor why the person hearing the no cannot say "I disagree with your answer, but I accept or respect your right to say it." The point is, if we commit ourselves to learning the art of saying no, we then must accept others' right to say no too, even when they give us no explanation for doing so.

We also need to remember that part of the learning to say no process is learning when and under what circumstances it is appropriate to say no without explanation. One of the most obvious situations in which it is inappropriate is when a patient asks for information concerning his health or health care. No without an explanation is appropriate in any situation that exists with peers, other professionals or loved ones when our primary reason for giving the explanation is based on fear, guilt or a sense of our own unworthiness. In essence, if our behavior is based on feelings of fear, guilt or low self-esteem, we cannot become autonomous. Inherent in the process of becoming autonomous is an element of risk that includes the risk of taking a chance on our own ability to say no — without fear, guilt or a sense of being unworthy. If we are afraid to take that chance, it is unlikely we will ever be able to say no anyway.

Implications of Saying No

In learning to say no, we must make sure we are aware of all its aspects. Certainly it is fun to fantasize about saying no to many of the demands that are a part of almost every woman's life, but the realization that others may not accept our new-found ability makes the fantasy less fun. Learning the art of saying no does not guarantee that significant others have also learned it or are willing to accept it from us; they may well withdraw their love and support, and the consequences can be extremely painful to us. No one likes to feel ostracized, unacceptable and unloved, all of which can occur because we have learned the art of saying no. Knowing about it and thinking through what our feelings and behaviors will be when it happens to us can mean the difference between successful completion of our search for autonomy or returning to passivity and dependence. If we always give in, if we are always the self-sacrificing martyr, if we continue to play the doctor-nurse game, we most assuredly will never see nursing become a significant force in the health care industry, just as we will never see ourselves become self-actualized persons free to respond with behavior that is not limited to the stereotypic behavior of the past.

Most human beings can work within a rational relationship that includes an occasional no without becoming angry, defensive and punitive. Many more of us can accept no's from others when they are given without being offensive and rude. There are ways of saying no that do not incite anger in the person being refused. Ordinary courtesy should certainly be a part of our ability to say no gracefully. Couple good manners with a firm but gentle tone, and many of our no's can be given with every hope of success. Success in this sense means that people respect us and respect our right to say no to a request. A successful no answer is understood to mean no to that particular request and does not imply that all

146 further requests will also be answered with no. A successful and appropriate no also means that the person giving the answer does not *have* to justify the answer to the other person. "If I feel I *owe* people my explanation, I will probably feel that I owe them my behavior as well, and then I will never be able to say No" [1].

When we learn to say no, we also learn to appreciate others' ability to say no to us. Once we have a good feeling about ourselves regarding saying no to others, we can perceive that they *honor* us by saying no to us. First, we can make the assumption that they feel we are reasonable, decent human beings who will respect their sense of self-esteem in having the ability to say no. Second, they apparently care something about us.

To illustrate this point: parents frequently must make the decision to say no to their children because to say yes would bring harm to the child. It may be argued that children make demands that are unreasonable and perhaps dangerous to themselves because they have not had enough life experiences to be able to choose wisely every time; on the other hand, adults, in making requests, know what is dangerous or injurious to themselves. Whether you agree or disagree that adults are able to choose wisely is not the point. The point is that many times, in saying no to adults, we say it for the same reason: it is not in the requester's best interest to be told yes. We say no because we care about the person making the demand.

An example may make the point more understandable: We have all met at least one nurse who is really a fine person and a good nurse, but who just does not have much sense of responsibility toward her job, her peers or the patients, particularly when she wants to do something else during the hours she is scheduled to work. Consequently, she feels free to ask others to work for her — to "cover her shift." Now, I may care about her as a person and respect her as a nurse and she may truly be a friend. If I always say yes to her demands, however, I am decreasing her possibilities for becoming a more mature, more responsible, more self-actualized person. By saying no, I am also saying it is in her best interest for me to say no to her. The same person will learn that my saying no to her request for me to work her shift does not mean that I am saying no to everything about her or our relationship. In fact, she will learn that I really think she is a fine person. If I always felt compelled to say yes, it would imply that she was a tyrant — a selfish, insecure, childish person who could not tolerate hearing no. That would mean that she was not my friend because I do not like selfish, insecure, childish people. She will also learn that because I can say no to her, I can also make demands of her, knowing that because she is under no obligation to me for having always said yes, she can also say no to me comfortably. If she says yes to me, it will be because she wants to and not because she feels she *owes* me a yes answer.

When a Nurse Should Say No
I have been discussing some of the reasons why people should and should not say no, as well as how we should say it and when it should be said. I have also talked about its relationship to our self-worth and others' perception of our worth. We now need to consider how the art of saying no relates to our self-concept as a nurse. For most of us, our sense of being a nurse is intimately involved with our sense of being a woman. It is difficult, if not impossible, to separate the two aspects of our *gestalt,* and probably totally unnecessary to do so. After all, we do not leave our *nurse* at work and assume our *woman* at other times. But the fact remains that nurses need to integrate the art of saying no into their *nurse* concept as much as anywhere else in their lives, if not even more. It is important for us to learn to say no to the unreasonable demands made upon us at work, just as it is important to say no to the unreasonable demands made upon us by society. As I have already suggested, we need to start with saying no to such things as demands to work for unreasonably low salaries, poor working conditions and little or no control over our own practice. We also need to learn to say no to our own impulses to be all things to all people. We need to learn to resist the temptation always to say yes to every request. Because we have been socialized as women to be the helpmate, support and coordinator of the home, we tend to assume responsibilities for groups of tasks and functions that are not directly involved with the business of providing care to our patients. The idea that much of nursing is not easily defined or measured tends to lead us and others into the trap of thinking that almost all activity in a health care agency is somehow related to patient care. And in

148 one sense that is true. After all, if the agency was not in the business of providing health care to patients, there would be no need for the agency; however, the fallacy lies in the belief that all patient care activities are directly related to the *nursing* care of that patient. There are many patient care activities, one of which is nursing. It is to our advantage as a profession, as well as in the patient's best interest, that we in nursing limit our activities to those things which are, in fact, nursing. Without the ability to say no, we will never be able to limit and define nursing in practice. We may be able to define it in theory, but others in the health care system either will not be cognizant of our definition or will choose to ignore it unless we also define it in practice.

The first step of the definition is our ability to say no to demands that keep us from practicing. The theory of nursing care involves the processes of assessment, intervention, implementation and evaluation. In current nursing situations, these activities encompass both simple and highly complex functions, any or all of which can be interrupted by other people's demands if we cannot learn to say no. For instance, the functions associated with assessment may range from the simple tasks of taking and recording vital signs to taking and recording an entire patient history. The accuracy and quality of assessments are crucial for effective patient care, yet we frequently allow others to interrupt us or keep us from making an assessment at all because we have not learned to say no. It is a sad commentary on our self-concept as a nurse when we are so busy with activities that are somehow related to patient care that we have no time to provide *nursing* care. Whenever I see a nurse who tells me she does not have time for assessments because she is too busy doing more important things, I begin to wonder about her capabilities as a nurse. If those other "important things" are in fact things that other health care personnel have decided are really nursing care because they are somehow related to patient care, I know that that nurse has not learned the art of saying no.

The next step in the nursing process is intervention. "At the lowest level, those tasks can consist of summoning the house doctor, making a bed, calling an aide for assistance, or discussing a patient with a therapist" [8]. Again, there is the nurse who does not know how to say no, who finds she is frequently interrupted as she cares for patients by others with "more important" tasks for her.

Consequently, she frequently relinquishes this aspect of nursing care to others with less skill. In many instances, the nurse does not perform even these low-level functions. At the very maximum, the nurse may see that the physician's plan of treatment is carried out. But in order for nursing care to be an important part of the total health care provided, nurses need to understand the significance of the highly sophisticated forms of intervention. Certainly, a part of intervention is interpreting the information garnered from a patient assessment. Interpretation is the ability to translate facts about the patient into concrete action. The concrete action may range from making sure others know the patient's likes and dislikes concerning food to the construction of a complex plan of care that involves several other disciplines. The fact is that the nurse can be involved in judgment and decision-making on a highly sophisticated level, but she must first have the ability to say no to other things and other people that will keep her away from involvement with the patient. In other words, you cannot make sound decisions based on hearsay. If the only information you have comes from other people involved in the patient's care, you cannot implement a plan of care for that patient that is based on good nursing judgments. We live in a highly complex, ever-changing world, and the field of nursing is no different than the rest of society. Nursing care is a dynamic process and nurses need to be aware that intervention is no longer limited to implementing doctors' orders. Today's concept of nursing practice includes the higher levels of clinical intervention that involve clinical competencies in nursing care that are crucial to a patient's recovery. If nurses cannot say no to all the extraneous demands that the health care system puts to them, however, they will never be able to intervene on any level but the most elementary one.

A part of intervention and implementation of most plans of care is instruction. Patient education has long been the purview of nursing, but in the fast-paced atmosphere of today's acute-care hospital setting, as well as in most ambulatory care settings, patient education is overlooked. It apparently is not considered very important by any of the health care providers, even though all of us give lip service to it. In many instances, physicians assume that nurses will do it, while nurses assume they cannot until the physician tells the patient his/her diagnosis. By the time that occurs, the physician discharges the patient without consulting with the nursing staff regarding patient education or any other aspect of the nursing care plan. The end result is that the patient goes home without knowing a great deal more about his/her health status than before admission and little or nothing regarding maintaining it. Is there any difference in an ambulatory setting? No. In fact many times it is worse, because we who work in ambulatory care have no more expertise in the art of saying no than nurses who work in acute-care settings. We also tend to make assumptions about the patient, what he knows and wants to know, as well as assumptions about other members of the health care team and what their responsibilities are toward the patient.

Probably our first assumption is that the patient's primary goal is to get in and out of the health care agency as quickly as possible. In many instances, that may be true. (Nevertheless, most patients spend more than an hour waiting when they visit any health care provider.) Second, we assume that the patient will not be receptive to efforts to teach him about health in general or his own health care in particular; however, this is false. In a variety of ambulatory settings, patients have been found to be highly receptive to health-teaching on a one-to-one basis or in small groups. As our society becomes better educated, individuals tend to want to know their own responsibilities for their health. They want to know about their bodies, how they work, how they respond to stresses, what they can do about preventing chronic health problems. The list is end-less, and the questions tend to force health care providers to stay alert and abreast of new developments in their field. This may be one of the reasons we do not offer health-teaching more often — we may be fearful that patients will force us to admit we are not as knowledgeable as we want them to believe we are. In effect, we are saying yes to our impulses to maintain a mystique about the provision of health care since it makes us feel powerful to know what others do not know. By doing so, we say no at the wrong time, for the wrong reason and to the wrong person. We need to be able to say no to people who waste our time at meetings where nothing is accomplished; we need to say no to interruptions from people who really have no reason to interrupt; and we need to say no to our own impulses that keep us tied to stereotypic patterns of behavior that are residuals of the past.

There are very few valid reasons why waiting rooms of ambulatory settings cannot be supplied with books, magazines and pamphlets on health instead of the latest movie, sports or news magazines. There are very few reasons why they could not also be supplied with audiovisual aids such as closed-circuit TV with "movies" that range from how to do a self breast examination, to what blood pressure has to do with the total state of health, to the safety hazards found in most homes. Most waiting rooms could be equipped with the necessities for health-teaching for not much more than the price of a good stereo sound system, which many of them have. We who provide health care, for the most part, totally neglect one of the most vital elements in the whole process, and nurses are as guilty as other health care professionals. We allow others to distract us from one of the most essential ingredients of the patient's recovery and maintenance of health when we do not say no to the distractions that keep us from teaching the patient about his/her own body and health. The nurses who work in ambulatory care settings also frequently make the assumption that the patient was taught all he needs to know about his health problem while he was hospitalized, and that it is the doctor's responsibility to carry the educational process along. Of course, neither assumption is valid. As nurses begin to assume responsibility for providing primary health care to people in ambulatory settings, they will discover that patients, given any opportunity at all, will seek them out as health educators. If we continue to say no to the patient instead of to the system that keeps us from providing nursing care, we have not learned the art of saying no, nor are we practicing nursing.

The last step in the nursing process is evaluation. Evaluation is measuring what we did against what the outcome is for the patient. In other words, we ask ourselves: "Did our plan work?" "Was it the right plan?" "Did we choose the correct priorities?" "What could we have done to make the plan more successful?" As we ask such questions, it becomes obvious that evaluation must begin at the time of implementation and remain a dynamic part of the nursing care we give. Frequently nurses never make evaluation a conscious part of their nursing care on any level or at any time except to make sure they have completed the day's tasks as demanded by doctors, administrators and other departments of the hospital. In reality, it is difficult to evaluate if you have not assessed the

152 patient, devised a plan and implemented that plan. If you have little or no base-line information about the patient, you probably cannot make sound judgments regarding his progress in recovering. By virtue of the fact that nurses cannot say no to others, we become so involved with other aspects of the health care situation that we have no time left to be involved with the reason we chose to be nurses — the patient. If more nurses can learn to say no, we will be able to see what the Lysaught report visualized as happening. There will be "striking changes in the levels of nursing; greater development of clinical specialization; and significant alterations in the reciprocal roles held by nurses and other health personnel, particularly the physicians" [8]. It is my hope that the change with the greatest magnitude will be the change in nursing behaviors. As we assert our right to say no, we will be asserting our right to practice *nursing* without the sense of fear, guilt and unworthiness that is presently connected with our saying no.

References

1. Close, Rev. Henry I. On Saying No to People: A Pastoral Letter. *Nursing Digest,* January/February 1975, pp. 49–52. Reprinted from *The Journal of Pastoral Care,* Vol. 28, No. 2, June 1974, pp. 92–98.
2. Brandon, Nathaniel. *The Disowned Self.* Los Angeles: Bantam, 1973.
3. Gold, Doris B. Women and Voluntarism. In *Woman in Sexist Society: Studies in Power and Powerlessness,* Gornick, Vivian, and Moran, Barbara (Eds.). New York: Basic Books, 1971.
4. Adams, Margaret. The Compassion Trap. In *Woman in Sexist Society: Studies in Power and Powerlessness,* Gornick, Vivian, and Moran, Barbara (Eds.). New York: Basic Books, 1971.
5. Waldman, Elizabeth, and McEaddy, Beverly J. Where Women Work: An Analysis by Industry and Occupation. *Monthly Labor Review,* U.S. Department of Labor, Bureau of Labor Statistics, May 1974.
6. Bardwick, Judith M., and Douvan, Elizabeth. Ambivalence: The Socialization of Women. In *Woman in Sexist Society: Studies in Power and Powerlessness,* Gornick, Vivian, and Moran, Barbara (Eds.). New York: Basic Books, 1971.
7. James, Muriel, and Jongeward, Dorothy. *Born to Win,* 2nd ed. Reading, Mass.: Addison-Wesley, 1973.
8. Lysaught, Jerome. *An Abstract for Action.* New York: McGraw-Hill, 1970.

6 The Image Shapers

Carol Spengler

Women have served all these centuries as looking-glasses possessing the magic and delicious power of reflecting the figure of man at twice its natural size [1].
Virginia Woolf

Our contemporary world could best be described as a fast-moving, ever-changing, fragmented, technological one. Because of the speed with which change occurs around us and the accelerated increase in information, we oftentimes feel overloaded or bombarded with stimuli. Social, political, economic and moral values are also changing at an accelerated pace. One of the basic concerns that seems to have grown out of all this is our ability to communicate with one another. It seems as though most of us are concerned with communication in one way or another. Perhaps this concern has come about because we feel further removed from one another than we once did. Our communication with others, regardless of the form it takes, is our way of "connecting" with them — of staying in touch with something that is familiar while most things around us are changing. Even our ways of communicating are changing and there are greater and more diverse means than ever before. In the past, direct communication was the only means. Then, as the world progressed and developed, new means of communication have also been developed. Communication expanded

156 from a simple verbal type to a written type and then to electronic communication. The various media that allow us to communicate on such a massive scale have had a significant impact on our lives and our society, and this sophisticated communication system affects everyone. An understanding of the special effect that it has on nurses and other women is crucial; therefore, this chapter will focus on the specific media that are involved in mass communication.

Mass Communication

To begin with, communication implies a two-way process that eventually results in sharing and understanding. As a process, it requires four important factors: a communicator, a message, a medium and a recipient [2]. Of the many different types of communication, the type focused on here will be *mass communication*. The institutionalized media that have been set up to communicate with people on a massive scale are the print media, such as magazines, newspapers and books, and the motion media, such as films, radio and television [3]. The main advantage of these forms is that they are the most effective way of disseminating information to large masses of people. The greatest problem with them is that the communicator is not sure "how" the mass audience has understood or interpreted the message. Merrill and Lowenstein suggest that the mass audience is anonymous, large, heterogeneous, scattered and ever-changing. Because of this, those who are communicators evaluate by intuition the effect of their message. They communicate to their audience on the basis of their own likes and dislikes to a great degree. They point out that polls, surveys and feedback give them some feeling about their audience, but: "In effect, they project their own biases on the mass audience" [4]. They further comment that because the mass audience is amorphous and ever-changing, projecting their own ideas is probably as good a way as any to handle the messages being sent out. This chapter will show how the most significant and degrading biases that are projected in all the mass communication media are those directed at women. The communication media alone do not shape the image of women in our society, but an interesting question is how much does it contribute to shaping and maintaining the stereotypic image of women?

The mass communication media could be considered social institutions, as they are structured social entities that are supposedly organized to perform definite functions for the public. They are by nature conservative. They are primarily set up to conserve the social heritage and to achieve goals through some kind of social conformity. Because social institutions have and exert great social control, they struggle to exercise and retain whatever control has been acquired and if possible to extend that power [5]. As individual social institutions, the goals of the communication media are varied. They are organized to inform and educate the public, to entertain them and to transmit messages of a diverse nature. To determine whether individual goals have been met, the communications media would have to find out if the message got through to the audience as it was intended. The only way to determine this is to conduct communication research. Many people agree that human beings are affected by the messages that they receive from the mass media, but not enough research studies have been conducted in this area to define effective and ineffective messages along with their positive and negative results [6]. It is therefore difficult to determine whether the message that is communicated is the cause or the effect. The messages could be merely a reflection of the present beliefs and ideas of the audience, or they could actually be the stimuli that cause the audience to believe or think in a specific way. To date, there is still no clear-cut answer to this.

In recent years, a great deal of criticism has been directed toward the media by consumers and nonmedia people. One of the greatest criticisms by the public is that the media have not been responsible to the public in that they have not, to any appreciable degree, conducted long-overdue scientific research that would show the effects of the media on society. In response to this recent public outcry, it seems that members of the industry defensively respond that it is the industry itself that should evaluate the effects of media. They feel that the lay public lack the necessary background and skill to enable them to determine what effects the media have and how the industry should change. Members of the media also use the argument that "freedom of speech" is in jeopardy when others evaluate, criticize and attempt to suggest how the media should operate. At the same time, of course, the various media are sending out critical messages on a daily basis regarding politics, the economy, our various institutions, other countries, individuals, etc. They are probably no more expert in all these areas than many of the consumers who feel justified in evaluating and criticizing the media. It is reasonable to conclude, as Merrill and Lowenstein have, that mass communication is everybody's business. They believe that intelligent, informed, constructive criticism can come from people who are not themselves a part of any of the media. The mass media "is too public, too pervasive, too powerful, to be left completely to the rather small group of media people who prepare and disseminate the messages" [7]. All consumers living in a free society have the right and obligation to evaluate and criticize any social institution whether that be the health care system or the mass media. It is our responsibility to do this because these institutions do have an effect on us and the quality of our lives.

Women as a group are justified in being critical of the communications media. The issue to be explored in this chapter is not whether the media create a negative image of women or merely "reflect" an already developed stereotype. The fact is that all the mass communication media exploit and degrade women. Although everyone in our society is affected by the media, the effect the media have on women is the greatest [8].

Printed Communication Media

I would like to begin with an evaluation of one of our oldest and most important forms of communication — the printed media — and I will attempt to show how these media treat and project nurses and other women. To begin with, the printed media have a wide appeal because of their "reviewability." The sound and motion media exist in *time,* whereas people can scan, read or review printed material at their own convenience and in many different places. Because of the permanence of the written word and its accessibility, the reader can reread or review such a communication if he desires [9]. However, written communications require more effort and imagination on the reader's part.

Newspapers

Newspapers are one of the cheapest means of communicating with a mass audience. Although the audience has diverse interests, most

newspapers offer a variety of information that people may choose
from to read. Thus, the avid reader who devours the newspaper from
front to back will usually find items that range anywhere from
world events to local advertising (including clip-out coupons)
to the daily comic strip. Regardless of whether or not the reader
chooses to read the entire paper or only special sections, it is apparent that the activities and interests of men have a greater priority
than those of women. For example, an inordinate amount of newspaper space given to the coverage of sports is male-dominated. The
pages of the sports section are replete with "action shots," head-
lines and article after article pertaining to male sports. There will
be pages and pages of reports of national, state and local sporting
events involving men, with large pictures interspersed throughout.
At the bottom of a page may be a short article about one of America's
outstanding women tennis stars, for example, and her upcoming
international tennis competition, and at that, only a portion may
be devoted to her tournament; the rest of the article doubtless describes the men's events of the same tournament. Another obvious
difference in articles regarding women in sports is the amount of
space devoted to a description of their physical attributes and attractiveness. None of the male athletes is described in terms of
appearance nor are their physical attributes mentioned.

When other activities of women are reported, they are usually
relegated to the "women's" or "family" or "society" sections of
the newspaper. It is noteworthy that these sections very often are
found toward the back of the newspaper, behind the sports section
and just prior to the advertisements. When women do display unusual achievements or success, the accomplishments are often compro-
mised by descriptive captions such as the "mini-skirted lawyer" or
the "female firefighter" [10]. This exemplifies the extent of sexism
in reporting, and this type of exploitation is not even subtle.

The front pages of a newspaper, where national and world events
are reported, clearly illustrate the male domination that exists
throughout the world. With few exceptions, all the events of any
significant nature are dominated by the decisions and power that
rest with men. Only a few women are involved in major, decision-
making roles. It is also obvious that violent acts committed on
or directed toward other human beings are the domain of men.
The front pages and, in fact, the entire newspaper demonstrate this.

The Image Shapers

The syndicated columns that feature views on national or international issues are almost all by men. Those written by women most often offer advice to the lovelorn, helpful household hints and other "female-identified" topics. The fact that the newspaper industry seems to be "by and for the men in society" is illustrated in several other ways: it is male-intensive in employment practices, beginning at the top level with the publisher, down to the local newscarriers, and it is male-oriented in its message and content. Some progressive newspapers are beginning to change, however, if only to a minimal degree. We now see young girls working as newscarriers, an area previously dominated by boys. Some newspapers have hired a few women in responsible positions, have women reporters and have changed their format to highlight the activities of women in a more equitable manner. The "help wanted" ads are not sex-linked, which provides women with a greater opportunity for competing in the job market. Unfortunately, newspapers that have made these changes are still in the minority.

Nurses as a group do not fare much better than other women when they are fortunate enough to be featured in an article. To begin with, frequently, when an article focuses on some aspect of health care, it is only the "medical" aspect of care that is highlighted. When nursing is the focus, often the traditional (and frequently outmoded) stereotypes are used to depict the role or activities of the nurse. Not long ago, an article on specific nursing issues appeared in a midwestern newspaper. The two pictures that accompanied the article were typical of the symbolic "staging" that is almost always used when depicting nurses — two nurses bending over a desk reading a record and another drawing up an injection with needle and syringe in hand. Rather than showing the nurse as she listens and talks with a patient, as she teaches the patient regarding some aspect of health care, or as she interprets the data collected from sophisticated monitoring devices, she is depicted as the lady in white who gives pills and injections or reads a record. It is no wonder the public often thinks of us as being capable of only standardized and regimented tasks that require little thought or feeling. When in a position to do so, we should take advantage of every opportunity to change this stereotyping in reporting.

Another irritating and common occurrence in articles about nursing issues is that the person interviewed oftentimes is not a nurse;

frequently, he is a physician or hospital administrator. It is interesting to note that very often in these situations, male reporters seek out other men to speak for and about nursing. The attitude of both groups is paternalistic and chauvinistic: the reporters, who perpetuate in this manner the myth that women cannot speak for themselves, and the hospital administrators and physicians, who believe that they are best qualified to speak for nurses. This is slowly beginning to change, however, because in some areas nurses are working actively to establish better communication with members of the news media. When this change takes place on a broader scale, we will become the rightful spokespersons for our profession.

Some of the distortions about nursing that occur in the news media are the direct responsibility of nurses themselves, however. The reporter who is assigned to write an article about a specialized subject should investigate the area carefully if he is not familiar with it. Responsible reporters do this; however, it is not realistic to expect that the reporter will be an expert on every topic he covers. It will therefore be incumbent on the nurse to effectively educate the reporter about nursing and to carefully review the contents of the article prior to publication, whenever possible. Nursing involves complex social interactions between people as well as the physical aspects of care. This is often difficult to define and explain to others, and nurses who are in a position to give this kind of information to a reporter sometimes do not take time to formulate their ideas carefully in advance. There are several possible reasons for this. Because nurses (like other women) have seldom been called upon to provide information to the news media, and since their opinions are not frequently highlighted, they are flattered by the attention. As a result, the article reflects their self-consciousness and timidity. There is almost a fear of being articulate and truthful. It is as though the nurse is so intent on playing a role of "kindly nurturer and protector" that she does not communicate her concerns and criticisms in a strong and self-confident manner.

A recent article focused on the new militancy demonstrated in certain parts of the country by nurses who are going on strike in an effort to establish a greater voice in health care practice. It was a disappointing article because only nursing administrators were asked for their opinions regarding local nurses' responses to such action. All the nurses interviewed, except one, spoke in platitudes regarding the nurses' feelings about their local work environment and satisfaction. The message in the article then shifted to a discussion of advantages in the area. The information was probably good public relations for the hospitals being represented, but it was also probably not at all representative of the opinions of the vast number of nurses working in the area. The fact is, there is abundant evidence that nurses are becoming more militant — and for good reasons: They are tired of their handmaiden role; tired of the arrogance of others who always speak for them; tired of feeling undervalued; tired of paternalistic attitudes that serve to keep them "in their place" and out of the policy-making domain; tired of the "game playing" that goes on daily in the work world; tired of sexism and stereotyping; tired of chronic exploitation as women and as nurses. These are the reasons they take a defensive posture in attempting to define their roles more fully as professionals and to convince themselves and others of their value and worth. This militancy is a very healthy sign. It means that at last nurses are developing an offensive posture in working for those things that are important to us and to our profession.

Where nurses have been successful in educating the interviewer, they have made possible enlightened articles regarding some aspect of nursing. A nurse was recently featured in a newspaper article that highlighted her expanded role as a nurse practitioner. The newspaper had contacted her and requested an interview. Having had negative experiences with distorted and inaccurate information in previous newspaper articles, she insisted on prepublication review and approval. She also insisted on seeing the accompanying picture that showed her with patients. The end result was a concise and accurate portrayal of her role and responsibilities. This article gave the public a better perspective of the diverse functions that nurses perform in health care settings. The only inaccuracy was in the headline, which described her expanded role as a "medical" role rather than a nursing role. She had explicitly defined the difference in the article but had not seen the headline that was to be used. (In the future, she will review *all* aspects of any report, including the headline.)

In order to change the image of nurses (and other women) in the news media and to ensure that we are allowed to speak for ourselves, we must become astute media-watchers. When articles or news features about our role and scope are unrealistic, we should immediately direct letters to the editor or publisher of the paper in question. We should encourage our colleagues to do the same. Only through the continuous and cooperative efforts of many individuals will a positive change come about.

Magazines

Magazines are another popular source of communication with a mass audience. Because of our average educational level and affluence in this country, there is a great demand for specialized publications on every subject imaginable and of interest to almost everyone. These specialized magazines appeal to individuals with common interests. They may range from scholarly journals to general publications that focus on hobbies or crafts. New magazines come on the market almost daily, it seems, and some fade away almost as fast. Until recently, the magazines directed to the mass female audience mainly supported the traditional female role; they focused on the latest styles in clothes, hair and make-up that would help the woman to groom herself in the latest fashion. Most fashions, of course, are designed by men and change yearly.

There are many magazines on the market to help the woman with her role of wife and mother. They provide information on decorating the home, preparing food, pleasing a husband, disciplining children, developing hobbies, etc. Until very recently, these magazines shied away from political and economic issues, feminist ideas or issues or topics that are considered masculine in nature. Other than professional journals geared to specific female-intensive professions or occupations, the magazines directed at the female audience have primarily focused on perpetuating the acceptable female roles. Women have been depicted in these magazines as physically attractive, stylishly groomed "Barbie Dolls" whose main interest is in maintaining attractive homes and preparing nutritious, colorful meals for well-adjusted, "well-mothered" children and well-satisfied husbands.

News magazines are certainly read by many women and could be said to have a wide audience appeal. Again, though just as with newspapers, most of the important news seems to be made by men, and as more women have come to read these magazines, they have slowly become aware of this fact. In 1972, the first issue of *Ms.*

magazine was published, and it focused on common concerns and issues related specifically to women in our society. We now have a number of new magazines that are directed to female audiences. These magazines have a much more diverse and therefore more relevant focus for the contemporary woman. For example, they feature information relating to political, social, economic and moral issues as well as domestic issues. Probably the most notable change evident in these magazines is that they not only assume women are intelligent, diverse individuals, and therefore present relevant information, but their development, writing and publication are in the hands of women. Because of this, we now have a greater number of women communicating with other women. Instead of reading only those publications that focus on the traditional feminine role, we now have the opportunity to read about a wider variety of topics that have important implications for us as women. More importantly, these issues are written from a woman's perspective. In the past, our perspective was not considered to be very important. We will doubtless continue to see an increase in the number of new magazines developed to deal with interests and concerns of women. As more and more women become aware of their common problems, they will continue to increase their communication with one another and to use the various media to do this on a broader scale. When women are given an equal opportunity in employment practices within the various communication media, the focus and content of publications directed to the general public will reflect a female point of view as well as a masculine viewpoint.

Nurses, like other specialty groups, have many common interests and therefore there are magazines and journals geared to these interests. Through these publications, the roles, concerns and problems relating to nursing have been appropriately identified and realistically described in detail. The rapid changes that are taking place within our profession, too, are well documented and reported in many of these specialty nursing journals, contributing to the updating and understanding of practicing nurses. Unfortunately, the audience that reads these publications are mostly nurses, as would be expected. The magazines that have a wide appeal to large groups of people are focusing on health care issues to a much greater degree now than formerly, although the focus is still primarily on the medical aspects of health care and the system of health care itself. Again, cure aspects rather than care aspects receive the greatest attention. Coverage for nursing, in this respect, directly parallels coverage for women in general, as medicine (primarily men's work) is highlighted more frequently than nursing (primarily women's work). The magazine industry, like the newspaper industry, is male-dominated, and therefore the content in many general publications is male-oriented.

Several of the most accurate and comprehensive articles concerning the nursing profession were published in 1973 in *Ms.* magazine [11]. The authors had obviously investigated the problems and concerns of nurses as perceived by nurses themselves, and the overview of nursing was realistic. It is important that a vast audience like the subscribers to *Ms.* magazine be accurately informed about various groups such as nurses. It is even more important that the general public, including many more men, be educated about our profession. As with other areas of the communication media, women in general and nurses in particular must use every available method to push for fair and equal representation.

Books
Books of all kinds have played a significant role in American society, as they have been one of our most important communication tools. Through books, we have provided a written record of our early development and history, and books have been used to provide background, to educate and to entertain a vast audience of people in our society. As our population, affluence and educational levels have increased, the publication of all kinds of books has correspondingly increased, at an incredible rate. With the acceleration of new knowledge in all aspects of life, there has been an increasing need to record and communicate our discoveries. Regardless of whether the discoveries made deal with technological inventions, scientific theories, changing social values, economic factors or political considerations, they are recorded and communicated to others through various types of specialized books. At the same time, people's interests and values determine the focus and content of the books that are published.

Because most Americans are exposed to various types of books from an early age, it could safely be assumed that this particular medium is probably one of our chief socializers. Both men and women have been influenced significantly by the information they have read in books, regardless of the type. In almost every kind of book, as with newspapers and magazines, women have been portrayed as inferior to men. Americans, both male and female, are exposed to this practice very early in life. Analysis of different kinds of books illustrates how the undervalued, inferior position of women in our society is defined and perpetuated.

To begin with, our first exposure to books is usually as a young child. Learning to read is surely one of the child's most exciting developmental tasks because it broadens his ability to communicate and to learn new things. Unfortunately, the female child will be given a different picture of her gender than the male child will be given of his. These sexual biases that are instilled in children through behavioral and social means are also recorded in books.

Not until the women's movement began were any significant scientific inquiries made regarding the sex-role socialization of children through picture books. As women have organized and have pushed for equal and fair treatment of females in all aspects of life, we are beginning to see evidence of greater interest in research that relates to socialization and its outcomes. Much of the research being conducted in this area is being done by female scientists. One such study, which was carried out by Weitzman, Eifler, Hokada and Ross, yielded some interesting findings. These investigators feel that picture books are a vehicle for the presentation of societal values to young children and therefore play an important role in early sex-role socialization. "Children's books reflect cultural values and are an important instrument for persuading children to accept those values. They also contain role prescriptions which encourage the child to conform to acceptable standards of behavior" [12]. In an effort to study how sex roles are treated in children's books, they chose several hundred picture books that had been identified as the "very best," since they were winners of the distinguished Caldecott Medal. Along with these, they examined three other popular groups of children's books [13]. The results of this study of prize-winning books revealed the following findings. Women were almost invisible and were underrepresented in the titles, the central roles, stories and pictures in all books sampled. Most books were about boys, men and male animals. When women or females were represented, they had insignificant roles and remained nameless and inconspicuous [14]. In fact, in almost one-third of the Caldecott books sampled, there were *no* women at all [15]. "Loving, watching and helping were among the few activities allowed to women in picture books" [16]. The implied message was that only by playing the traditional female role can a girl triumph. "Women who succeed are those who are unobtrusive and work quietly behind the scenes. Women who succeed are little and inconspicuous — as are most women in picture books. Even heroines remain 'invisible' females" [17]. In the world of picture books, the activities for boys are quite different from those for girls. Girls are passive while boys are active. Boys are depicted in more adventuresome, exciting roles that illustrate more independent behavior as they pursue more varied activities. Girls, on the other hand, are depicted as passive and immobile. They are found indoors more often performing activities that up-hold traditional feminine roles. Boys are portrayed as leaders while girls are "servers." Self-confidence and independence are almost exclusively depicted as male attributes. "Little boys rescue girls or helpless animals" [18]. It is almost never the other way around. Through their varied adventures, boys are encouraged to develop a sense of camaraderie with each other while girls are rarely pictured working or playing together. "The role of most of the girls is defined primarily in relation to that of the boys and men in their lives" [19]. The stories imply that women cannot really exist without men. In regard to clothing, girls are frequently pictured as pretty little dressed-up dolls who are not meant to be active; they are to be admired and to bring pleasure to others.

When adults appear in these stories, they exhibit stereotypic behaviors. Again, men are active; women are passive. "When men lead, women follow" [20]. The most interesting and provocative finding was that there was *not one* woman who had a job or a pro-fession in the stories sampled from among the Caldecott books. This is ludicrous; as has already been pointed out, almost half the people working today are women. In these books, motherhood is presented as a full-time, lifetime job consisting of unrealistic and unchallenging tasks. For example, mothers are almost never

168 shown outside the home (i.e., driving a car, etc.) and are usually pictured as performing only household tasks and services for the father and children. Even these roles are depicted in an unrealistic manner. On the other hand, the father works outside the home and rarely helps with mundane housekeeping or child care [21]. Men are shown in a variety of interesting occupations. Occupational roles described for boys are very different than those for girls. " . . . the ultimate goal for which little boys are to aim is nothing less than the president of the nation. For girls, the comparable pinnacle of achievement is motherhood!" [22]. Girls and women are portrayed in the stories as dull stereotypes while boys are clever achievers. Girls are praised mainly for their attractiveness. Most of the women shown had achieved status on the basis of their relationship to specific men — not on their own. Both male and female characters reinforced traditional sex-role assumptions. Boys are to grow up to be intelligent and brave while girls are to grow up to be compliant and pretty [23]. Instead of being a stimulus for fantasy, achievement and imagination, these stories have served as a means for perpetuating basic cultural values and myths, which interferes with the "growing demand for *both* girls and boys to have a real opportunity to fulfill their human potential" [24].

Other studies have demonstrated similar findings. By the time children reach school age, they have already been bombarded with information that pressures them to adapt to sexist roles [25]. This does not stop, either. Textbooks used in schools depict men and women in much the same way. At the same time, boys are encouraged to cultivate an interest in those subjects that are traditionally considered masculine (math, science, etc.). Literature and history textbooks, regardless of grade level, exhibit two dominant patterns. "Either women are present in dating, mating or mothering roles, or they are totally absent" [26]. History books are probably the most notorious for evading reality and the significant role that many women have had in helping to develop and shape the destiny of early America. To read most history books, one would wonder why women existed at all except to perpetuate the human race through their reproductive functions. Young girls, studying the history of our country, will find very few strong role models to identify with because the accurate presentation of the significant contributions made by our female ancestors has yet to be written.

I am hopeful that this will change in the near future, as a number of historians (mostly women) are beginning to retrace our American history to point out the important contributions made by women. The myth that only "white males" struggled to develop America is now being challenged by others as well; black people, Mexican-Americans, American Indians and other minority groups have made contributions that history books have ignored. That these groups are not represented does not substantiate the notion that they played no crucial role in our nation's heritage. We have ample evidence that each of these undervalued and powerless groups was, in fact, exploited in one way or another by white males.

Women, for the most part, do not fare much better in fiction than they do in nonfiction. Wendy Martin retraced the image of women in American fiction and concluded that "heroines of American fiction have reenacted Eve's fall from grace and thereby inherited the legacy of Eden. As daughters of Eve, American heroines are destined to dependence and servitude as well as to painful and sorrowful childbirth because, like their predecessor, they dared to disregard authority or tradition in the search of wisdom or happiness; like Eve, they are fallen women, eternally cursed for eating the apple of experience" [27]. In many of our classic novels, women are characterized as subordinate, dependent weaklings who cannot tolerate being rejected by men. When women do break out of their traditional roles, they are severely penalized. They become fallen women who are shunned by society, or they die or they lead a dismal existence — or else they devote themselves to some noble task to exonerate themselves.

Seldom is the woman in fiction a strong, successful character in other than the traditional feminine role of wife and mother. When the woman is depicted as strong and successful, she is also presented as coarse and hard. A strong, masculine character then sets about the task of "taming" the shrew. A variety of means are used to do this, ranging all the way from simple tongue-lashings to exotic bedroom scenes where every sexual tactic including rape is introduced. Eventually, the woman will succumb or be outfoxed by the superstud masculine type. She will come to her senses and chuck her career or whatever important project she is involved in and will settle into marriage — her final reward. When the female character does remain strong and independent and does not succumb to the enticingly desirable male, it is implied that she is incapable of loving and will therefore lead a successful but lonely, desperate life. But these strong female types are not portrayed as often as the helpless, sweet, ultrafeminine creatures who search for (and find) their identity through male characters. The paperbacks provide us with many examples of this.

When the fictional female character is presented as the successful wife and mother, she is usually respected and beloved. This is because she is nurturing, supportive, compassionate — and sometimes "all knowing" as she serves her children, husband and community. The strength in her character is represented in her unselfish giving to others. It is not usually because of her unique individualism.

So — in fiction woman is a stereotype: a sex object, a fallen woman, a martyr, a kindly mother or a cold, calculating conniver. Of course, male characters are not always presented in a positive light, either. This unreal picture of women renders half of our population less than human. "Sacrificing the humanity of slightly more than 50 percent of the species is a pretty high price to pay for eating an apple — and it was probably a rotten apple at that" [28].

Fiction that is written to inspire and entertain potential nurses certainly needs a new type of heroine. Since the early 1930s, there have been many books that feature nurses as heroines. Lucretia and Elizabeth Richter reviewed 25 books on nursing in the young people's section of several public libraries. Their investigation revealed that such books are misleading and outdated — and indeed fiction! [29]. The most popular and best known heroines are probably Cherry Ames and Sue Barton. There have been many volumes of the *Cherry Ames* series since the early 1930s, but they have not kept up with the times — they are still back in that era. "Cherry and Sue attend training schools, learn to rise when a doctor enters the room, and memorize the procedure book" [30]. Interestingly, professional commitment is given less emphasis than is romance.

Then there are the many paperback and hard-cover nurse-romances. In reviewing these books, the Richters found that the central theme is for the young student nurse to meet and marry a young doctor [30]. In many of these books, the realistic daily challenges and drama that are inherent in the nurse's work world

are often missing. The challenging aspect of "catching a doctor"
seems to be the major theme. Interesting aspects of caring for
patients are sometimes presented (along with an abundance of
romance), but frequently they are inaccurately portrayed. Another
prevailing theme is extreme dedication and servitude. Often, the
characters are portrayed as feeling that they must inevitably make
a choice between marriage and nursing after graduation [30]. The
students are typically shown as having to work long, hard hours,
often alone, with a great deal of responsibility, or under the harsh
supervision of other nurses. They solve problems by instinct alone.
They are not independent, creative and intelligent people who
function effectively as a member of the health care team. The
setting, the role and the character of the nurse heroines are unrealistic and outdated. "Nursing is in its very nature full of drama,
excitement, tragedy, suspense and humor — all the natural ingredients of absorbing fiction. Among the thousands of American
nurses there must be many who could use these elements to entertain and inspire our nurses of the future" [31].

Some groups are taking aggressive steps to rectify the situation
of the female stereotype. The American Federation of Teachers,
AFL-CIO, passed a women's rights resolution in 1972 which states
that "teaching materials that portray limiting sex role stereotypes
can result in irreparable psychic damage and distorted aspiration
levels of women. Females should be portrayed more often as
'problem solvers, creators, and executors of ideas.' They should be
depicted in a greater variety of actions showing them as 'independent,
competent, athletic, persistent and interested'" [32]. They pointed
out that males should also be represented in a wide variety of activities including homemaking and child care. In family relationships,
individuals should not be portrayed as subordinate to others on the
basis of sex [32]. The union was serious when it adopted this
resolution. Not only did members commit themselves to the idea
of correcting sexist stereotypes in teaching materials, but they also
went a step further. They notified educational publishers that they
would not purchase their books until the sexist portrayals were
changed [32].

While women in many books, even at the present time, are presented as rather weak characters, our true strength is starting to be
recognized — even though begrudgingly. The growing impact of

the feminist movement is beginning to be felt. A major book publishing company has recently established "guidelines for the equal treatment of the sexes." The guidelines begin with a definition of sexism and go on to explain that the company is attempting to eliminate sexist assumptions from their publications. They also state that through these guidelines they are trying "to encourage a greater freedom for all individuals to pursue their interests and realize their potentials" [33]. There are eleven pages of recommendations for nonsexist treatment of reference works, teaching materials and other nonfiction. Prior to the feminist movement, this kind of recommendation would not have existed. It is interesting to speculate on whether the pressure was brought to bear by the American Federation of Teachers or other pressure groups, or if some form of legal action was the precipitator. Certainly, without the constant efforts of many women and some men, changes in relation to unfair treatment of women in the publishing industry would not be occurring. We have a long way to go, but we have made a strong beginning. Our progress will easily be traced and recorded through the written media of the future!

The Electronic Media

While the printed media have increased our means for communicating with one another, their impact cannot be compared with that of the electronic revolution which has had a tremendous effect on culture and politics throughout the world.

Shortly after radio and television were discovered, a high degree of message saturation was achieved. And our lives have not been the same since. Radio is now available to almost everyone — not just in affluent America but in many remote villages around the world as well. I recall traveling in the Middle East, in sparsely populated villages where the majority of people were illiterate, but radios could be heard everywhere. News events from other parts of the world were reported regularly and were interspersed with local happenings and music. It was strange to be far away from the United States and yet remain so well-informed about important current events.

Radio and television, of course, have a great potential for teaching. At the same time, they can perpetuate illiteracy, because it is now so easy to receive news without having to learn to read or to make any effort other than looking or listening [34]. Merrill and Lowenstein point out that "the electronic media also have great potential as multipliers of democracy. At the same time, they exist as powerful instruments for authoritarian control" [34]. Merrill and Lowenstein suggest keeping in mind the fact that both radio and television are susceptible to government control and both are basically entertainment media. Because of government regulations regarding appropriate and "positive" conduct, radio and television are under closer surveillance than the printed media [35], being regulated through their local stations by the Federal Communications Commission (FCC) [36]. Through the FCC, these stations are granted a license to broadcast for three years at a time. In order to receive a license, the stations must operate "in the public interest, convenience, and necessity" [36]. The FCC has defined many rights that belong to the people, and if a station does not follow the guidelines, it will lose its license to operate. (This fact should be imprinted on the minds of all women for future reference.)

Radio and television function primarily as entertainment media because they are especially appealing to the eye and ear. Also, little effort is needed in order to take advantage of them. Their tremendous potential is not being fully utilized in educating and informing the public. This seems to be of little concern to a large segment of the average public, however [37] — and national surveys bear this out — the exception being the news programs, which are primarily "guests" in this entertainment world [37]. The mass audience tolerates some time devoted to news, but their main interest is in being entertained. To be convinced of this, one has only to recall the furor that occurred when the "Watergate" hearings were televised daily. For the first time in American history, pre-impeachment proceedings against a president were being debated and televised, but many viewers were angry and critical because the televised hearings interfered with the game shows and soap operas. A compromise was eventually worked out so that each day a different network televised the hearings, causing fewer interruptions in the regular daily programming. The public could then choose between the hearings and their regular entertainment.

Television came into being during the 1940s along with many

The Image Shapers

174 other significant technological developments. Alice Embree has pointed out that this new mass medium developed quickly as another giant profit-making corporation whose chief influence has been to "shape people into one-dimensional receivers of communication" [38]. She also identifies the mass media along with mass education as the "chief socializers of young people, the chief value-setters and image-creators" [39]. Opponents of this idea would say that we do not have sufficient scientific data at this point to validate these theories. On the other hand, as has been pointed out already, human beings are affected by the values and behaviors that are promoted and reinforced within their culture. Television certainly promotes specific values and behaviors through its programming content. When one considers that almost all Americans have at least one television set, regardless of their economic background, and that many spend a major portion of their relaxation time watching television, it is only reasonable to conclude that this particular medium must take credit for influencing and therefore shaping the image of Americans to an increasing and significant degree.

"A child between the ages of three and 12 who is a 'moderate' television viewer spends more than 1000 hours a year in front of the tube — more time than the child spends with a teacher, or in many cases, with a parent" [40]. Teachers and parents are acknowledged as having important, long-lasting effects on educating and socializing children. Any child who spends the same amount of time with the electronic babysitter as he does with a teacher or parent must be significantly influenced by it!

Television was credited with serving an important purpose when it brought the Vietnam War into the living rooms of millions of American homes; presented special documentaries on overt acts of discrimination directed toward blacks and other minorities (not women); highlighted examples of environmental denigration and pollution; identified sources of political corruption and criminal acts such as "Watergate"; and pointed out other social ills of the day. If television can be credited with influencing public opinion on these issues on a massive scale, it can only be concluded that it is just as capable of influencing people in negative ways.

Entertainment television characterizes all human beings as ridiculous and foolish, but, typical of the entire communication

world, it particularly exploits women. "Women are constantly
presented as passive, submissive, vain, empty-headed sex objects,
incapable of rational action and conscientious only about their
roles as wives and mothers" [41]. These stereotypes are repeated
over and over on television, from the commercials through the entertainment programs. Because this negative image of women is
so all-pervading on television, we are consistently robbed of our
human dignity. These stereotypes have been perpetuated for so
long that they seem believable and natural to many people. A large
number of women have been thoroughly proselytized into believing that the emotional, nonthinking role assigned to women and
projected consistently on television is their natural role. For many,
this form of "mind control" has been so pervasive and complete
that they are not aware of its dehumanizing aspects and their
subsequent oppression.

Where does it all begin? At the beginning, of course, which leads
us to the organizational control of television. Television, like the
rest of the communication media, is male-dominated. The executives
of most stations, from the national to the local level, are men. Less
than 7 percent of all radio and television announcers are women
[42]. Seventy-three percent of the writers, artists and entertainers
are men [43]. Since they have the major control administratively
within the media and since the majority of writers are men, they
should be credited with the creation of the content involved in
programming. It is easy to see why so much of prime-time programming is devoted to the male-oriented world (i.e., police and
detective stories, westerns, etc.). Doctor and lawyer shows are
quite popular now and almost always feature a male lead. Where
women are present, with few exceptions, they play subsidiary
roles that perpetuate traditional stereotypes. When a woman is
the star of the show, she is often assisted by or relates to a male.
Some attempts to change this have been pretty weak. For example,
in one series, the star is an attractive blonde policewoman who is
capable of handling a gun very well. She is daring and courageous
and oftentimes goes overboard. Her male partner, along with the
rest of the masculine crew, is always quick to the rescue. Sexual
innuendoes usually are present in the script. This program can be
given some credit, however, for projecting a woman in a non-
traditional role. Since police stories and violence seem to be

The Image Shapers

favorites of male audiences, it appears that the only real change was to add a respectable sex symbol to another boring but violent story.

"A study of characters in network programming (other than commercials) showed that of 1,830 portrayals, 81 percent were male, 18 percent were female" [44]. These statistics speak for themselves. An evening of television viewing would demonstrate the same results. A few shows that attempt to deal with the lives of contemporary women are beginning to be aired. Various groups, such as the Image of Women Committee of the National Organization for Women, are partially responsible. This group monitors the communication media and sponsors a variety of activities aimed at upgrading the image of women in the media.

Another area of television in which women have had minor roles is in newscasting. In the past few years, however, a new breed of journalists has developed — young, articulate, well-educated, personality-laden, photogenic female television reporters [45]. As Connecticut Walker has pointed out, "No TV station can afford to be without one" [46], and all networks feature them now. These women do a competent job and measure up to their male colleagues very well. The question that Walker has raised pertains to the criteria women reporters must meet in order to become television journalists. Are youth, personality and good looks, along with competence, essential prerequisites for female TV journalists? When one considers the current group, it is fairly obvious that they *have* these characteristics. Will they be put out to pasture when they become middle-aged? It is also obvious when one considers the personal characteristics of male television journalists that they have not had to meet the same kinds of prerequisites. Some network executives deny that beauty and youth are major requirements for women. Others feel that women's talent is important, but if two equally qualified women are to be considered for the job, the more attractive one will get it [46]. Connie Chung, CBS network correspondent, states "the networks are reluctant to put ugly women on the air whereas they use a number of men who are fat, bald, or not very handsome" [46]. The double standard reflected in network hiring practices partially results from the fact that television viewers are more critical of the appearance and personal characteristics of women reporters. Related to this, "many women TV reporters feel that their femininity, their looks, their figures prevent them from being taken seriously, that these characteristics detract from the substance of their reporting" [46]. Audiences seem to be overly conscious of the visual image presented by these reporters and are therefore more demanding of women than of men. This is often reflected in the mail or phone calls that female reporters receive. Some stations are also more demanding regarding the visual image of women reporters in that they require women to conform to specific standards regarding their hair, make-up and wardrobe [46]. Women have, however, made some progress regarding employment in television newscasting.

Since television is primarily viewed as an entertainment medium, a variety of different programs is offered. Over the past few years, there has been a growing interest in health care, which seems to be reflected in the large number of programs that focus on this. The image of women, and nurses in particular, that is projected on these shows is typically unrealistic and negative, however. Daytime programs are geared more to women, since women make up the major portion of the audience and the daytime programs are therefore different from nighttime programs, which are geared to the male audience. Regardless of the time of day, however, nurses and other women are presented in a disparaging manner.

In the daytime, interspersed among game shows, situation comedies and kiddie programs, are the "soap operas." The themes of two popular soap operas that are viewed with regularity by an untold number of women deal with multiple, complex and often unrealistic interpersonal conflicts among the characters. Few of the female characters are depicted in professional, productive roles. The only ones who are treated so are the female physicians — and there are not many of those. The image and role of the professional nurse is that of a scheming, conniving woman whose main goal in life is to trap a doctor. Besides the focus on the marriage game, there is little else to illustrate the challenges and responsibilities faced by real nurses on a daily basis. The nurse is usually depicted as a submissive, unintelligent, often unfeeling robot who rarely makes a move without a doctor's order. This is carried to such extremes that one is given the impression that nurses are not capable or allowed to function at all without directions from a physician. In addition, the nurse is rarely ever found at the patient's bedside.

The Image Shapers

178 She is chronically at the nurses' station with her symbolic tools: the chart, the telephone or the typewriter. She is rarely, if ever, portrayed as a competent, assertive, intelligent, caring human being who has equal but different responsibility for the health and well-being of those who are cast as patients. When she is not portrayed as a robot, she is cast as emotional and hysterical, the implication being she is a woman and this is the way women are.

Another type portrayed is the immoral nurse. This is the woman all other women most fear because she is the "marriage crasher" — the woman who is out to get another woman's man. She will use any means to attain her goal, including those that are inherent in her situation as a nurse.

As in any group, there are nurses who are not competent, intelligent, responsible or strong. But this is not true of the majority, as the media would have the public believe. People are already disillusioned with inadequate health care, and watching just one of these absurd soap operas would do little to reassure them when they need to rely on a professional nurse for any aspect of their health care. Also, this type of programming perpetuates sexist attitudes among youngsters who may be watching. It could certainly encourage a young person who is contemplating a career in nursing to look elsewhere.

Evening television entertainment is more of the same thing. It is, however, a bit more sophisticated, as it also has a larger audience of men. There are a number of medical shows that dazzle the audience with the latest electronic devices and equipment, dramatic medical maladies and handsome heroes with superhuman powers to resolve problems. The hero, of course, is almost always the physician, and to make the picture complete, nearly always is male. Some relevant social issues are dealt with, but as usual, all work out in the end on a positive and often unrealistic note. There are many female nurses shown, but male nurses do not usually appear in any of these sagas. The image of the nurse on evening programs is slightly different from that seen on the daytime soap operas, the most common characterization being a young, pretty, breathless, big-breasted, long-haired, mini-skirted, high-heeled, sexy cretin! She is technically competent when the physician dramatically barks directions, or she is silently in the background doing little or nothing, waiting for her next command. The entire milieu is one of high drama, precision efficiency at the command of the physician, technological paraphernalia, stiff formality among all characters (except the patient and physician), and an attractive but insignificant nurse. Sexual innuendoes directed at the character of the nurse are not uncommon.

Another characterization of the professional nurse is that of a rigid (and probably frigid) middle-aged, surly, army-sergeant type who is ill-tempered. She has been around a long time and is recognized as being experienced. She has a strong, assertive personality and often knows "what's best" but instills fear in student nurses and young doctors. It seems from all this that the nurse is never portrayed in a strong or important role unless she exhibits negative traits. She becomes the archetype of the aging, nagging or domineering woman. This characterization is one way television has of putting women down. The other nurses in the story, of course, do not like the army-sergeant type nurse, and this is often illustrated in the form of negative remarks and disapproving looks behind her back. The younger nurses ally themselves with the physicians, who also disapprove of the aging nurse. Occasionally, when her suggestions are heeded and it turns out that her solution was right, she will be thrown a crumb of recognition by the super-specialist young doctors.

The portrayal of the nurse as a competent, compassionate, responsible professional who is skilled in resolving either routine or complex patient care situations is rarely given. Instead, she is the proverbial chart-carrier who responds to orders in an automatic way and seldom interacts with patients in any meaningful way. In the real world of health care, the nurse is often a heroine, for her astute observations and quick action can make the difference between life and death. In less dramatic situations, the nurse's actions may be significant to the patient's recovery, rehabilitation or adjustment to illness. In numerous situations, a nurse's actions and reactions have been the deciding factor in preserving a human life. On many occasions, the nurse's personal relationship with a patient has made a difference in his coping with or adjusting to an illness. The majority of nurses, given the opportunity, could relate numerous such experiences. Knowing the real world of nursing as I do, I become angry when I view the prostituted image of professional nursing that is projected by the television media.

The public is much more sophisticated and knowledgeable concerning health care than in the past, and as intelligent human beings, they should be presented with a more realistic portrayal of the professionals who provide care for them. All the workers composing the health team have special skills that are necessary in providing services to patients. Each group should be valued for its unique contribution. Unfortunately, because of the medical shows, the myth is perpetuated that the physician is the single most important person providing health care. This myth exploits the other health care workers, especially the nurse.

Elaine Beletz conducted a research project in which she studied how the public perceives nursing today. Her results showed that the public views the nurse in the same way that they did in the past — in sex-linked, task-oriented terms [47]. The group she surveyed were hospitalized patients who were fairly young (aged 18 to 39), primarily white, and middle-class, with a nearly equal distribution of males and females. It was interesting to note that everyone in the study group had had some prior personal contact with the nursing profession, and most of them indicated a familiarity with medical television programs [48]. When asked to describe what they witnessed the nurse doing on television and what they had actually seen her do or thought she did in the hospital, "taking doctor's orders, giving medications, serving meals, carrying things about, giving shots and providing bedpans" were the answers [49]. Although the patients in this study stated that television does not portray nurses accurately, they, in fact, perceived nurses as functioning in much the same way as television portrayed them. Beletz concluded from her findings that the influence of television is perhaps a subtle one. "The role of the nurse that people see presented on television may sensitize them so that they immediately identify similar functions they see in actual practice and remain oblivious of unfamiliar functions" [49].

The television media are beginning to get the message that women want fair, positive portrayals of women and the issues that concern them. Recently, a number of specials dealing with women's issues have been shown during prime viewing time, and there are several new weekly programs that focus on sensitive and important feminist issues. The disparaging image of women as presented by the television industry is *slowly* beginning to change. Why? Because various organizations and groups are filing petitions with the Federal Communications Commission in an effort to prevent license renewal to those stations that continue to downgrade or debase women. Also, complaints are being filed with the FCC regarding discriminatory employment practices in the industry. With all these efforts combined, it is possible that in the future, when we flick on the television, we will see women portrayed in roles that give recognition to their varied interests, activities and potentials. Only when this occurs on a broad scale will the image of women be one that reflects their human dignity.

Films

There are 8 women and 3,060 men in the Producers' Guild. Twenty-three females and 2,343 males are members of the Directors' Guild. There are 148 women and 2,828 men in the Writers' Guild [50]. These figures shed some light on why women are projected as they are in films today. The film industry is no different from any of the other communication media. It too is male-dominated and projects women in unflattering and sexist roles in the majority of movies. Molly Haskell, a sharp observer of movies and a film critic, has traced the movies and how they have portrayed and betrayed women from the early 1920s to the present time. She contends that "movies are one of the clearest and most accessible of looking glasses into the past, being both cultural artifacts and mirrors" [51]. Future generations who flick on the late, late show to see the old reruns from our present decade will see women presented in demeaning and dehumanizing roles. Since the beginning of the film industry, the role definitions accepted by society have been reflected in microcosm in films. Interests and activities for men and women are different and opposed to one another. The man is supposed to drive himself to create, to achieve and to conquer. He is more himself when he does this. When he is reflecting or making love, he is least himself. Woman, on the other hand, is more herself when she is in the throes of emotion. When she pursues knowledge or success, she is not considered to be womanly. Haskell points out that a "movie heroine could act on the same power and career drives as a man only if, at the climax, they took second place to the sacred

182 love of a man. Otherwise, she forfeited her right to that love"
[52]. In most movies, women have not been allowed to sacrifice
love for a career. For the most part, the portrayals of women in
films have merely perpetuated traditional roles and functions.
This has been done, however, in a highly romantic and unrealistic
way. To some degree the traditional roles have been glamorized,
perhaps to make them more palatable to the audience. In a sense,
Hollywood has served as "the propaganda arm of the American
Dream machine" [53]. Haskell points out that "the anomaly
that women are the majority of the human race, half of its brains,
half of its procreative power, most of its nurturing power, and yet
are its servants and romantic slaves was brought home with
peculiar force in the Hollywood film" [54]. Actresses who became great stars invaded the dream lives of other women and helped
to shape the way they thought of themselves. These actresses
embodied many stereotypes when they played roles of love god-
desses, martyrs, mothers, spinsters, virgins, broads, prudes, vamps,
she-devils, adventuresses and sex kittens [55]. In the film industry,
during the 1920s, 1930s and to a lesser degree in the 1940s,
actresses reflected, perpetuated and sometimes offered innovations
on the roles of women in society. There were some stars, however,
who were independent-minded, strong individuals and who were
cast in roles that demonstrated their strength and character. "Here
we are today, with an unparalleled freedom of expression and a
record number of women performing, achieving, choosing to
fulfill themselves, and we are insulted with the worst — the most
abused, neglected and dehumanized — screen heroines in film
history" [55]. For the past ten years film portrayals of women
have been the most disappointing in the history of the industry.
Films have moved from covert misogyny, to kindly indifference,
to overt violent abuse and brutal treatment [56]. The great roles
for women of our decade that will be recorded for history are
mostly those of whores, emotional cripples, sex-starved spinsters,
losers, psychotics, space-brains, castrators and drunks. The women
featured in the 1960s and 1970s are less intelligent than before,
less humorous, less sensual and less extraordinary [57]. It seems
that over time, as women have moved closer to becoming liberated
as human beings, they have been projected in the movies in more
demeaning, sexist, dehumanizing roles. There have been only a

few films that have depicted women in more spirited, stronger roles. In the future, the film industry, like other institutions, will have to present women in more realistic, valued and humanistic roles. And women will have to lay the groundwork for this. "It becomes imperative for woman to reinvent herself, to create an identity that is not just an inoculation against 'falling in love' but that exists transcendentally for its own sake, and that will eventually enable her to go beyond herself to the world at large, to an interest in its history which she at last will have a hand in shaping" [58].

In movies, nurses have been characterized similarly to the way they and other women are portrayed on television. They frequently play an insignificant role, standing in the background waiting to "run and fetch" for others. And sometimes the nurse is presented as a sensual siren who is a ready bed partner for patients, the medical staff and just about any other male available on the scene — hardly a positive image. Women everywhere must work together to break through the barriers of our commercial cinema. Sexism in technicolor is one of the more obvious ways of putting women down.

Advertising and the Communication Media

"The influence of advertising is so pervasive that one has difficulty in clearly identifying its role in mass communication" [59]. Some argue that advertising should not be a part of the media, and others feel it is necessary to maintain a competitive free-enterprise system. The important question is, what role does advertising play in the communication media and how does this subsequently affect nurses and other women?

To begin with, many of the television programs are free because advertising subsidies pay for them. The cost of magazines and newspapers is less because advertising reduces the cost. The other communication media, such as books and movies, somehow survive without advertising within or on the actual product [60]. These do rely on other advertising, though, because without it we would not know what books are available or what movies can be seen. Other media are used to advertise books and movies, so in a sense it cannot be said that any of the media could survive without some form of advertising. Merrill and Lowenstein point out some

184 interesting facts about advertising. Approximately two-thirds of the daily newspaper revenue is income from advertising. Sixty to 75 percent of the average daily is devoted to advertising; therefore, the reader pays less but also gets less reading matter. They also point out that much of the expense to the consumer of newspapers and magazines is incurred because of advertising functions. Taxpayers subsidize newspapers and magazines by paying additional federal taxes to have them delivered by second-class mailing rates. Taxpayers also pay to dispose of these products after they are used. The television viewer pays for free programs by being forced to spend 15 to 20 percent of his viewing time watching commercials. It seems safe to say that there is no such thing as completely free television. Approximately 80 percent of the commercial income from networks is derived from products such as deodorants, beverages, soap, cosmetics, toothpaste, patent medicines, hair products, breakfast foods, etc. Interruptions in programs to insert advertisements pertaining to these products are frequent and often irritating to the viewer. At least in newspapers and magazines, the reader can choose to look at them or not and does not waste his time on advertisements that are of no interest to him [60].

Does advertising control the media? Yes, but not necessarily in a direct way. In reference to the print media, advertisers are concerned with the "audience" as opposed to the "message." "Indirectly, advertisers control the content of the print media they subsidize, since the publications attempt to attract an audience that will be most satisfactory to current and potential advertisers" [61]. It is not the social indispensability of the newspaper that makes it survive but rather the ability to attract advertising [61]. The advertiser is concerned with both the audience *and* the message in the electronic media. Advertisers insist on sponsoring specific programs rather than specified numbers of hours of general advertising. Because of this, the advertisers' product or name becomes closely linked with the program. They therefore prefer to sponsor programs that will be popular, will be shown frequently and will attract mass audiences. The advertiser's influence is negative rather than positive. If a program is controversial or does not have wide appeal, advertisers will not want to sponsor it because they might not sell as much of their product. Since the major goal of businesses and corporations is to make a profit, those things that interfere with this will be eliminated. Networks hesitate to lose advertising revenues; therefore, other than the news and some specials, few controversial programs are aired. It would be too costly. This inverted relationship of advertising to program content influences the type and quality of programs viewed by the audience. Even though this influence is indirect, it is still a controlling factor over the media. Merrill and Lowenstein have pointed out that advertising is merely a message, not a medium, and it is therefore responsible only for the content of the advertising message and not for the program in which it appears. The media, on the other hand, are responsible for the message content they send out to the mass audience. As long as the media allow advertisers to dictate which programs and what kinds of programs they will sponsor, in essence they will be controlling the program content given to the public. The communication media functioning in a free society are responsible for preserving truth. The media are regulated to a degree by the government. Advertising must also be regulated to prevent misleading and unfair practices. Advertisements and commercials that are offensive, misleading and too frequently or inappropriately placed between programming should be strictly controlled [62]. The television industry has been irresponsible in this area as it continues to increase the number of commercial minutes allowed per hour instead of adequately increasing the rates for advertising.

If the media are responsible for the message content sent to the audience, it would stand to reason that any message sent through those media would also be their responsibility. This is not true and most networks announce that they do not endorse products that they advertise. This whole area seems like a double message for the audience. Stations say, "We do not necessarily endorse these products" and then they provide advertisers with inordinate opportunities to interrupt program viewing time with messages about products "they don't endorse." Through the FCC, consumers can bring about changes in unfair programming and hiring practices. The FCC obviously does not or will not attempt to control advertising appropriately. As a result, consumers, especially women, continue to have their viewing interrupted by absurd commercials that are frequently insulting; these disruptive commercials do exert considerable influence on the viewer, however.

For example, one study of prime-time network commercials showed that women were revealed as "decorative sex objects." In 32 percent of the commercials, there was no real message and in another 20 percent they represented wife/mother characterizations. Women were conspicuously absent in commercials pertaining to executives, lawyers, scientists, professors and athletes [50]. In another study, which reviewed 986 commercials, 43 different occupations were represented for males and only 18 for females, including housewife, which made up 56 percent of all the commercials. Also, 38 percent of the females were shown inside the house while only 14 percent of the males were. Women were between the ages of 20 and 35 in 71 percent of the commercials and only 31 percent of the men were this young. Women, when they appear at all, are typically pictured as young housewives, at home, demonstrating some product used in the bathroom or kitchen. When women are shown out of the home, it is most often in a service role such as that of a secretary or stewardess. Advertisers consider the male voice to be authoritative as opposed to the female voice, and this is shown clearly by the fact that women's voices are heard in only 6 percent of the commercials [63]. All one has to do to determine what advertisers think about women is to spend a few hours watching television or leaf through any well-known magazine or newspaper. The message is the same as that put out by the communications media. Women are emotional, neurotic, vain, empty-headed, dependent people whose primary concern is keeping a clean house, buying and preparing food to please husbands and children and making themselves over to look younger or more attractive to others. Their portrayal in advertising is the same as it is in children's books, texts, newspapers, magazines and television programs. The theme is consistent. Obviously, advertising is not being properly regulated or the misleading, offensive practices that are used in attempting to promote products would cease. Most advertising devalues women and perpetuates them in stereotypic, sexist roles. A great deal of money is spent by corporations for advertising purposes. It must pay off or they would choose other methods of selling. But women are in a good position to change this situation, as they are the major consumers in this country and can boycott those companies that persist in exploiting women. They can also write letters of complaint to magazine editors, television networks, newspapers and advertisers themselves. The Image Committee of NOW monitors ads on radios and television to show evidence of sexism and then initiates action with advertisers and broadcasters. They also present anti-awards yearly to the 40 advertisers who present the worst image of women in television commercials. Advertising ethics are questionable at best. Selling a product is their main concern, not the integrity of the message. Since advertising has not controlled its own industry to any appreciable degree and does not seem to be overly concerned about the tactics used to entice people to buy, outside groups, including the government, should develop standards for their policies. These should then be monitored and enforced. Those advertisers who do not comply with appropriate standards should be properly penalized.

Advertising directed at nurses unfortunately is not much better than that directed at other women. When nurses are shown in advertisements, they are portrayed in stereotypic and sexist roles. The professional role of the nurse is confused with the sex role of the nurse. Some of this advertising takes place in our own professional journals. The editors in a sense endorse the exploitation of nurses as women by allowing the sexist and demeaning type of advertising that is found throughout the classified ad sections.

Another type of advertising that is commonly seen is the kind that attempts to appeal to the nurse by giving a romantic description of the area in which the hospital or agency is located. For example, one advertisement reads:

Philadelphia — city of brotherly love, city of tradition, city of change! Now undergoing a dramatic renaissance, Philadelphia will see more exciting changes in the years to come . . . and you can be part of it all! As a staff nurse at the Hospital of the University of [X], you will work in a complex medical center in the heart of this dynamic metropolis . . . minutes from orchestra concerts, pre-Broadway theatre, famous stores, museums, and historic shrines . . . Convention Hall and other sports centers are steps away. And being part of a great university, you may enjoy the stimulating academic life. A tuition refund plan is available. Shouldn't you find out more about the way of life that awaits you here?

I am sure that for most of us, the place we choose to live reflects our cultural and social interests to some degree. This advertisement covers information pertaining to those aspects pretty well, but what does it say about nursing? Nothing much! A good travel agency could provide all this information and probably cover it in more depth. This type of inappropriate advertising related to professional nursing must end. To continue to allow it to be used to "lure" nurses to employment settings is irresponsible on the part of our profession. We should certainly be able to establish acceptable guidelines in our professional journals regarding advertising practices. Failure to do this will make us accomplices in our own exploitation.

So, in both advertisements in magazines and commercials on television where the nurse is portrayed, a traditional, stereotyped role is depicted. The nurse is in the background somewhere, in full uniform, doing something insignificant like reading a thermometer, perpetuating the traditional and outmoded image of the nurse. Just about everyone can take a temperature, including the nurse. The fact that most nurses spend very little time, if any, carrying out this task demonstrates how far behind the advertising practices are. This also demeans our profession. Society will never view us in a more realistic and positive manner unless we work together to change those false and inappropriate practices in the media and in the advertising industry. We also need to become media-watchers and initiate aggressive action against those who have not attempted to upgrade the image of nurses. Our professional associations should work closely with such groups as NOW. Whatever happens to women in general is also reflected in the treatment of nurses as a specialized group. Our profession needs to develop a well-organized public relations program that will inform the public about the diverse and expanding roles of nurses. Other educational programs, seminars or conferences geared to the consumer should be carried out on a nationwide basis. In carrying out these activities to improve and increase the understanding regarding the role of the nurse, we would also be doing something constructive for women as a whole. The men in our profession would benefit too when the image of nursing is projected in a nonsexist role.

Perhaps one of the most difficult and yet most important changes that will have to take place in order for the image of the nurse to improve is the attitude and behavior of nurses themselves. If nurses have high standards for their own practice and that is made visible to the consumer through first-hand personal experience, a greater understanding of what nurses actually do will develop. Emerging from this will be a realistic and respected image of nurses and of other women as well.

It should be remembered that "the simple mirrors that hang over bureaus and on the backs of closet doors only tell us super-ficial physical things about ourselves. The real-life mirrors are the media, and for women the most invidious mirror of all is advertising" [64]. It should take little to convince us that the image of nurses and other women, as projected in the media and advertisements, is shallow, demeaning and unrealistic. When we are given an equal opportunity to live and develop as full human beings in a "free" society, the distorted image of women will be corrected. It is the women in our society who will bring about the needed political, economic and social reforms necessary to make this a reality. And many women are already hard at work!

References

1. Woolf, Virginia. *A Room of One's Own.* New York: Harcourt, Brace and Company, 1929, p. 60.
2. Merrill, John C., and Lowenstein, Ralph L. *Media, Messages, and Men.* New York: David McKay, 1971, pp. 6–7.
3. Ibid., p. 11.
4. Ibid., p. 13.
5. Ibid., pp. 92–93.
6. Ibid., p. 138.
7. Ibid., p. 157.
8. Embree, Alice. Media Images I: Madison Avenue Brainwashing — The Facts. In *Sisterhood is Powerful,* Morgan, Robin (Ed.). New York: Vintage Books, 1970, p. 181.
9. Merrill and Lowenstein, op. cit., p. 48.
10. National Organization for Women, Image of Women Committee, New York Chapter. Images of Women in the Mass Media, (pamphlet) p. 2.
11. Kushner, Trucia D. The Nursing Profession: Condition Critical, and Fleeson, Lucinda B. Doctors Diagnose Nurses. *Ms.,* Vol. 2, No. 2, August 1973.
12. Weitzman, Lenore J., et al. Sex-Role Socialization in Picture Books for Preschool Children. *American Journal of Sociology,* Vol. 77, No. 6, May 1972, p. 1126.

13. Ibid., p. 1127.
14. Ibid., p. 1128.
15. Ibid., p. 1129.
16. Ibid., p. 1130.
17. Ibid., p. 1131.
18. Ibid., p. 1135.
19. Ibid., p. 1136.
20. Ibid., p. 1139.
21. Ibid., p. 1141.
22. Ibid., p. 1144.
23. Ibid., p. 1146.
24. Ibid., p. 1148.
25. Maccoby, Eleanor. Sex Differences in Intellectual Functioning. In *The Development of Sex Differences*, Maccoby, Eleanor (Ed.). Stanford, Calif.: Stanford University Press, 1966, p. 26.
26. Howe, Florence. Sexual Stereotypes and the Public Schools. In *Women and Success*, Kundsin, Ruth (Ed.). New York: William Morrow, 1974, p. 126.
27. Martin, Wendy. Seduced and Abandoned in the New World: The Image of Women in American Fiction. In *Woman in Sexist Society: Studies in Power and Powerlessness*, Gornick, Vivian, and Moran, Barbara K. (Eds.). New York: Basic Books, 1971, p. 329.
28. Ibid., pp. 345–346.
29. Richter, Lucretia, and Richter, Elizabeth. Nurses in Fiction. *American Journal of Nursing*, Vol. 74, No. 7, July 1974, p. 1280.
30. Ibid., p. 1280.
31. Ibid., p. 1281.
32. Doyle, Nancy. Woman's Changing Place: A Look at Sexism. *Public Affairs Committee, Inc.*, No. 509, June 1974, p. 6.
33. McGraw-Hill Book Company. Guidelines for Equal Treatment of the Sexes in McGraw-Hill Book Company Publications.
34. Merrill and Lowenstein, op. cit., pp. 63–64.
35. Ibid., p. 66.
36. Ross, Susan. *The Rights of Women*. New York: Avon Books, 1973, p. 149.
37. Merrill and Lowenstein, op. cit., p. 67.
38. Embree, op. cit., p. 176.
39. Ibid., p. 180.
40. Choate, Robert B., and Debevoise, Nancy M. Battling the Electronic Baby-Sitter. *Ms.*, Vol. 4, No. 10, April 1975, p. 91.
41. National Organization for Women, op. cit., p. 1.
42. Sommers, Dixie. Occupational Rankings for Men and Women by Earning. *Monthly Labor Review*, U.S. Department of Labor, Bureau of Labor Statistics, August 1974, p. 39.
43. Ibid., p. 37.
44. Doyle, op. cit., p. 21.

45. Walker, Connecticut. Newswomen and Television — Beauty on the Tube. **191**
    Parade, February 16, 1975, p. 4.
46. Ibid., p. 5.
47. Beletz, Elaine E. Is Nursing's Public Image Up to Date? *Nursing Outlook,*
    Vol. 22, No. 7, July 1974, p. 432.
48. Ibid., p. 438.
49. Ibid., p. 433.
50. Doyle, op. cit., p. 20.
51. Haskell, Molly. *From Reverence to Rape — The Treatment of Women
    in the Movies.* Baltimore: Penguin Books, 1974, p. xiv.
52. Ibid., p. 4.
53. Ibid., p. 2.
54. Ibid., p. 3.
55. Ibid., p. 30.
56. Ibid., p. 323.
57. Ibid., pp. 327—329.
58. Ibid., p. 368.
59. Merrill and Lowenstein, op. cit., p. 79.
60. Ibid., pp. 83—89.
61. Ibid., p. 85.
62. Ibid., pp. 87—88.
63. Doyle, op. cit., pp. 20—21.
64. Komisor, Lucy. The Image of Woman in Advertising. In *Woman in
    Sexist Society: Studies in Power and Powerlessness,* Gornick, Vivian,
    and Moran, Barbara K. (Eds.). New York: Basic Books, 1972, p. 304.

7   Politics of Power

Marlene Grissum

*Those who have real power over our lives recognize the threat we pose —
even when we ourselves do not [1].*
Robin Morgan

Perspectives of Power

The very word *power* produces anxiety and a sense of conflict in many women and, consequently, in many nurses. Instead of hiding our heads in the "sands of status quo," we need to start examining the whole concept of power and our conflicts about it. Some understanding of power and its use is essential in order for nursing to grow as a profession or, for that matter, even to maintain its present position in the health care system.

Our power as nurses probably lies in the fact that the society in which we live recognizes nursing to be an essential service, even though individuals within that society cannot define nursing, nor, in most instances, do they know *why* it is an essential service.

Jo Ashley contends that "nursing power, as a productive force, is the single most important factor maintaining our health care systems today. Without the pooled energies of individual nurses, health care facilities across the nation would be forced to shut down or offer a far different kind of service than they do at present" [2].

There are two main perspectives of power: the "influence per-

193

194 spective" and the "social control perspective" [3]. We in nursing need to learn about these and to understand them, both their use and their implication. According to Gamson, the definition of "influence" used in this sense is the "intended effects of actors upon the decisions of other actors." Social control perspective looks at the use of power as it relates to "the ability of a society to mobilize and generate resources to attain societal goals." Both of these can be means to exert pressure on those in the health care field who now hold power and authority over us.

Conflict, an integral part of seeking power, is oftentimes seen by women as too costly a price to pay for power. They fail to see conflict in its more positive aspect, that of a catalyst — an opportunity to achieve a power base and thereby establish a means to increase their influence on our society. Gamson contends that "the ability to handle conflict successfully is a critical leadership skill" [3]. Perhaps women, and nurses in particular, should be aware that they lack leadership skills when they reject an opportunity to effect change because the conflict involved in power changes is too uncomfortable or anxiety-producing for them to handle.

"All politics, all leadership and all organization involves the management of conflict" [4]. If Schattschneider's statement is true, the next question that must be asked is: "How has nursing managed conflict in our health care system up to now?" The answer seems to be that we have been the mediators. This idea agrees with Gamson's theory on conflict regulation. He says that "in a pluralistic social structure with the presence of multiple, overlapping group memberships, the structure of such groups serves to encourage compromise. The existence of overlap between groups creates a peculiar circumstance: the boundary of one group is a potential line of cleavage in another. A conflict between two overlapping groups cannot be pressed to the fullest by either group without running the risk that it will create a breach within itself. *Those who belong to both conflicting groups are natural compromisers and mediators*" [italics mine] [3].

If one looks at the health care system as a "pluralistic social structure," it is easy to see why nurses fall into the trap of being the compromisers and mediators. There are many nurses who see themselves as members of the group called medicine; these same nurses see themselves as part of the group I will call hospital administration; and also they see themselves as members of the group called nursing. If, for instance, a conflict of power arises, as it frequently does, between medicine and hospital administration over patient care policies, nurses are the natural mediators, since they and the others involved perceive nurses as belonging to both medicine and hospital administration. Neither medicine nor hospital administration can press the conflict too far because both can lose what they both need — patients. But both can look upon nursing as the mediator because nursing not only needs patients, but it also needs hospital administration — to provide work space, equipment and supplies — and medicine — to provide patients. In the final analysis, what usually happens is that nursing is left holding the bag. Nursing, by being the compromiser, agrees to some policy that medicine has declared they would not do but hospital administration has declared must be done. For instance, most hospitals have rules set by the administration regarding how often doctors see hospitalized patients. The hospitals I am familiar with require at least one visit daily, which must be recorded on the patient's chart. Frequently, in the nurse's notes you will see the notation "Doctor here." There will be no note made by the physician. This note made by the nurse is a tradition now, but in the beginning it was a compromise by the nurse to maintain the legality of the record for the benefit of medicine and hospital administration. The nurse filled the gap between the physician, who was too busy to write a progress note, and the hospital administrator, who declared that a note must be written in order to make legal charges to the patient for the physician's visits.

Nurses are also compromisers with other sectors of the hospital hierarchy. Nurses become pharmacists in many hospitals after midnight, nurses become lab technicians after midnight and on weekends (particularly in ICUs, where blood gases, electrolytes, etc., need to be drawn frequently), nurses become physicians after midnight and rationalize all such behaviors by saying that it is for the good of the patient! Nurses have become compromisers within the hospital system to the extent that they have allowed nursing procedures to become a complete mystery to the public so that the average patient has little knowledge of what nurses do other than take orders. As a result, the public does not recognize nursing care as separate from medical treatment.

Politics of Power

If nursing power does lie in the fact that society recognizes nursing as an essential service and if the average patient has little knowledge of what a nurse does, what does that say about our power base? It says our power is built on weak and shifting sand, and this should be changed as quickly and efficiently as possible. If patients do not know what nursing has to offer them, how do they know they need it or want it? And how is a nurse going to be able to prove to patients or third-party payers that it is worth paying for?

Let us see if there are ways Gamson's two main perspectives of power can be applied to our situation in order to achieve the power nursing needs to maintain control over our profession.

The social control perspective looks at the use of power as it relates to the ability of a society (nursing) to attain its goals. If our goals are to attain power over our own profession, to practice autonomously, to be accountable and responsible for the nursing care we give, we must start by exerting the inherent power we have against the health care system we have. Needless to say, there will be conflict and there will be struggle. Neither should be unfamiliar to nurses, however. Our very history began with a power struggle. Florence Nightingale fought the whole health care system and the whole system of male supremacy in order to start an educational system for nurses. Down through the years there has been the struggle for education, the struggle to assert ourselves as a profession and the struggle to practice nursing as nurses have defined it, not as others have defined it. Finally, all of us have struggled with the need to define nursing to ourselves and others, and to convince others of its value and its importance to the health care system. So, the struggle must go on; at least that part of our conflict will be familiar to many of us. But other aspects will be totally alien and thereby frightening as we pursue, isolate, confront and examine power and the way in which nurses need to use it.

In a study done on the success-failure rate of social groups trying to bring about social change, Gamson [5] found that there were several factors involved in successfully bringing about desired changes. His data seem appropriate for nurses to understand and use as we strive for changes within the system we so confidently call health care. One very interesting piece of data is that violence oftentimes leads to success! One of Gamson's definitions of success is that the group gained new advantages for its constituents and beneficiaries and accomplished its goals. "In the case of violence, it appears better to give than to receive if you want to succeed in American politics" [5].* None of the nonviolent recipients of attack met their goals. Violence is even more successful according to these data "when the group goals are limited and when the group does not aim to displace its antagonists but rather to coexist with them" [5].*

Violence is not the only kind of pressure that can be exerted to bring success. Eight out of the ten groups studied that had used such methods as strikes, boycotts and efforts to humiliate or embarrass their antagonists were successful in bringing about acceptance of their group and new advantages for their group. Gamson presents the idea that violence or force, such as strikes, is the product of confidence, impatience and a rising sense of power rather than frustration, desperation and weakness. The groups he studied that were successful in their attempts to change the social order were large; only one had fewer than 10,000 members. "Such numbers seem more likely to breed confidence and impatience rather than desperation" [5].*

Another important aspect of Gamson's research, as far as nursing is concerned, is that "a group needs a bureaucratic structure to help it become ready for action, and centralized power to help it reach unified decisions" [5].* The three prerequisites listed as necessary for a bureaucracy are: "It must have a constitution or charter that states the purposes of the group and rules for its operation... It must keep a formal list of its members... It must have at least three internal divisions, e.g., executives, chapter heads, rank and file" [5].* Centralization as defined by Gamson is when "power resided in a single leader or a central committee, and local chapters had little autonomy" [5].* Some of the groups he studied had centralization without bureaucratic organization; some had bureaucratic organization without centralization but: "Groups that were both bureaucratic *and* centralized had the best chance of achieving their goals; 75 percent of them were successful" [5].*

How can we in nursing who are advocating change and assertion of power use this research to gain our goals?

*Reprinted from *Psychology Today* Magazine, July 1974. Copyright © 1974, Ziff-Davis Publishing Company. All rights reserved.

Perhaps we had better look first at our professional organization, as well as our professional feelings about achieving success. In other words, are our goals real and do we want them badly enough to take the risks involved? Does our professional organization have the characteristics listed by Gamson as necessary for success? Can we apply these concepts, which were written about American political groups, to a group that is not political in the sense of politics, but needs to be political in the sense of attaining and using power? Will the professional organization be the bureaucratic, centralized command post nurses need or will it bow out of such behavior, crying nonprofessional?

First, does it have the correct characteristics? Yes, it does have a constitution, it does keep a formal list of members and it does have at least three internal divisions.

Second, will it bow out? That is very doubtful. The ANA has supported nurses all across our country who have struck for better pay, better working conditions and/or control over nursing practice. With that kind of background, it seems unlikely that it would bow out now, particularly in view of the fact that it has also publicly announced support for the Equal Rights Amendment, and continues to give evidence of listening to the demands and wishes of its constituency at the Biennial Convention. The fault, if there is one, lies with the rank and file who do not voice their wishes to the leadership. We need to be explicit, to give the leadership the mandate to organize our professional organization along the guidelines set out by Gamson. We need to make sure every member understands that our goal is to achieve power over our own destiny and what methods we are going to use to achieve that goal. If nurses are really serious about gaining the power of nursing for nurses, we should start to consider what methods have been successful in the past for what groups and use that information in order to be successful now.

Gamson defines a group as centralized if power resides in a single leader or central committee, with local chapters having little autonomy. Any nurse who is a member of the ANA knows that our professional organization does not meet Gamson's criterion for a centralized group. If the constituency so desired, we could mandate that the ANA become so centralized.

This call for a strong, centralized professional organization smacks of unionism, it is true, but we need to explore the idea to see if there is a way to use it to our advantage.

To start with, our professional nursing education has socialized us to believe that professional people do not form unions, that it is not professional, that we do not need unions because we are dedicated to a higher cause. In retrospect, it seems that because we have continued to believe such myths, we have let one of our chances to control our own destiny slip away. What, after all, is a union but the joining together of a group of people with similar work interests who have more power as a collective than they would have as individuals?

It is unfortunate, at least from a power base point of view, that modern nursing developed beside modern medicine, because that fact alone, according to Ashley, accounts for many of our difficulties. "Medicine obviously has more recognized power than nursing. However, medicine has not always been so powerful, and would not now be so powerful, if the medicine profession had not managed to control, limit and use the power of others — notably nursing — to strengthen its own" [2].

Medicine was able to control, limit and use the power of others, at least partially, because physicians were a highly organized group that worked as a group to reach their goals. The power of medicine in contrast to the power of nursing is a commentary on the male-female roles in our society. Those stereotypic views need to be changed *now* in order for both medicine and nursing to provide quality health care for consumers in this country. It is time for medicine to stand on its own power and to stop using nursing power to help legitimize its control over the health care industry. It is time for nursing to start asserting its power for the benefit of nursing rather than for the benefit of medicine. "Nursing is not and never has been medicine; this fact needs to be better understood by nurses, as well as by physicians and the public. Our power now and in the coming decades should be devoted to changing attitudes — especially the one that sees nursing as simply a vehicle or means of producing that which physicians wish to dispense in the name of health care" [2].

If, in the process of changing those attitudes, one method is unionizing into a powerful, cohesive group with enough political clout to be heard above the babble of self-named authorities in

200 nursing, what matter? We will not be the first professionals to form such a group (not that being first is bad) nor will we be the last. We need to recognize and cultivate the power we do have and then use it in an intelligent and logical fashion. Our ability to practice, *at all,* in the future may well depend upon it.

Perhaps it is disconcerting to find nurses who advocate such drastic changes — that have no idealistic views on professionalism — who are willing to join other nurses in a strong, cohesive group to attain power over their own practice and over nursing as a profession. But I contend that nursing has finally matured — we are no longer the sweet, innocent teenagers of the health care system. Instead, we have reached a mature, level-headed, realistic adulthood. Our idealism has grown into the realism of experience. We *know* what we must do in order to achieve success. We must assert the power given us by society and use it to provide the essential service we owe them for having given it to us. "A successful group is one that is ready to fight like hell for goals that can be met without overturning the system" [5].*

There is another aspect of power that we need to explore, but in order to do that I must first digress and spend some time investigating what Elizabeth Janeway calls "social mythology" [6]. If we are intent upon changing attitudes and behaviors within our own profession and within the other health care professions with which we have relationships, we must begin to understand where attitudes and behaviors come from, what influences them to change or remain static and how people begin to believe and accept attitudes and behaviors as their own. Janeway [6] says that "we understand who people are only in terms of what *we think* they *ought* to be" [italics mine]. In other words, we prescribe a set of attitudes, actions and behaviors that help us to define and understand who people are. To sociologists, we are defining a role. A role is a dynamic thing — it must have action — so we are actors.

Talcott Parsons' definition of "role" is "the aspect of what the actor does in his relationship with others seen in the context of its functional significance for the social system" [7]. To put it more simply, it involves activity, relationships and a social system.

Attitudes and behaviors are our own reflections of our self as

reflected back to us from the significant others in the relationships
we develop within our own social systems. In order for our attitudes
and behaviors to be acceptable to ourselves and others, both
parties — the *role-player* and the *role-other* — must share an understanding of the meaning of the role.

Now, there are other forces that impinge upon a role besides
the role-player's own attitudes and behaviors about her role and
the expectations and responses of the role-others, those who help
us define our role. But they are all inextricably woven together to
assist us in our performance. As long as our performance is good
(i.e., what people expect), we are assigned that role. But if our
performance is bad (unexpected or changed behavior), people
no longer understand — they become threatened or frightened —
and we are looked upon as a deviant; one no longer able to perform
that role. We have become a "role-breaker" [6].

Perhaps that is what is happening in the relationships of nurses
and other health care professionals. We are no longer performing
the role of nurse as we once did and as role-others still believe we
should. What others think we ought to be and what nurses think we
ought to be are no longer the same. We are no longer willing to
play the role as it always has been played. So physicians, hospital
administrators and other health care personnel are threatened;
they no longer feel safe in their own roles because they no longer
feel they know the right responses to make as a role-other as
far as nurses are concerned. And so we hear "What do nurses
want?" Now, this is the same question we hear, as women, in our
role as women — "What do women want?"

I believe that Janeway's quite simple explanation serves as a
beautiful and succinct answer for both questions. "Women want
control over their own lives and authority or influence commensurate with their abilities in the external world" [6]. In other
words, we want the power to control our own destiny, not
necessarily power to control others.

According to Janeway, social myths are the "product of profound emotional drives, drives that are basic to life." Sometimes
they "substitute for action a will to believe that what they desire
exists — or should exist" [6]. We are all familiar with social
myths; we just do not call them that. They are the *everybody
knows* facts that make up our everyday language and behavior.

202 For instance: Everybody knows woman's place is at home, even though over 40 percent [8] of the work force are women! Everybody knows that women are passive, dependent, intuitive creatures who cannot be trusted, even though there are women who behave in aggressive, independent, analytical ways and hold responsible positions in our world. Everybody knows that nurses do not make decisions and act on those decisions; they wait for others to make decisions and tell them what to do, even though many nurses act decisively every day in all areas of health care agencies and in their own private practices. Everybody knows there is not much need for women to get higher education because they will never put it to use; they will just get married and stay at home. After all, everybody knows you don't need a college education to just be a housewife and mother, even though "2/5 of the married women in the United States hold jobs; more than half of them are mothers of children under 18 years old and more than 1/5 are mothers of children under six" [6].

These, then, are some examples of my understanding of a social myth. They are a circuitous route taken to reach another of our social myths — the female power myth. This is the myth that is the basis for much of the fear men express concerning women outside *woman's place*. As we begin to explore mythical power — particularly as it relates to women — we should bear in mind what Janeway says about myths, that they "remain attached to the emotions of those who uphold them . . . they gain strength from the connection that they supply to their believers . . . they endure because they offer hope, because they justify resentments, but perhaps most of all because they provide a bond of common feeling . . . Prove it false a hundred times, and it will endure because it is true as an expression of feeling" [6].

If a myth has all that going for it, including the idea that you cannot change it by proving it false, is there any necessity for or hope in trying to discuss the fallacy of the female power myth? I believe there is. When a myth affects the world of reality, it is because those who believe in it act to make it come true. Perhaps there are ways that those who do not believe in it can act so that it does not come true. With that in mind, let us look at the myth of female power and then at what we as women and nurses can do so that it does not come true.

Anais Nin says, "I have a feeling that man's fear of women comes from having first seen her as the mother, creator of man" [9]. Others, including Janeway, agree with her. "The myth of female magical power certainly had its origin in a period when the mother was the only parent, when her impregnation was as easily attributed to the wind, or the dew, or an ancestral spirit, as to the man she lived with" [6]. Mother is the all-powerful, all-seeing entity that provides everything for every want or need, even without our asking — sometimes before we even know we need it or want it. Because she is all-powerful and all-seeing she also has the power *not* to provide everything we want or need, because her power is absolute and continuous. "She can mold [her child] and shape its habits, play with it, tease it, teach it and frustrate it, push it toward fulfillment of her own desires and mock her husband's hopes, if she wishes to" [6]. Now, of course, in order for this power to be used, there must be two parties involved — the giver and the receiver — the child to demand, the mother to give. Without both parties, the power disappears.

There is an analogy here that nurses should begin to think about as we press forward in our search for freedom and autonomy and for control over our own professional lives. I will touch only briefly upon it now because it could be another book. The basis of the analogy lies in our giving — if we give good nursing care, i.e., what the doctor orders (wants), we are strong and powerful and rule our domain. We lose that power once we assert ourselves as thinking individuals who can decide for ourselves what good nursing care is — i.e., what the patient wants/needs — and set about doing it. In other words, we remain powerful as long as it is "private power in return for public submission" [6]. As long as we play the doctor-nurse game and let the physician have credit for being the one who knows what good nursing care is or should be, our illusion of power will be maintained.

Now, back to our myth about female power. If the positive side of the myth is the omnipotent mother — all-powerful, but all-giving — the negative side of the myth is the witch — the bad mother — according to Janeway. The witch is the part of the mother that abuses the mother's omnipotent power, that punishes us when we are bad, that thwarts our wants by saying no, that will eat us if we express too much anger or frustration. In other

204 words, a witch is a mother who has become a deviant; she no longer plays her role as prescribed.

In order to view this mythical female power in action in the present world, we need to look at both men's and women's behavior as it relates to women having or getting power. Let us look at the men first. Of course, we have to remember that myths are plausible and they "endure because they offer hope, they justify resentment" [6].

Who gets called a witch in the field of nursing? For the most part, it will be a title for nurses who question the system, those who never hesitate to question reasoning behind physicians' orders, those who demand more money, better working conditions, more control over their own profession, those who are not intimidated by ogres (the only negative role given to men — an exaggeration of the dominant male) [6]. In short, my definition of a good nurse!

Who does the name-calling? Both men and women. Men, for a variety of reasons that certainly includes their fear that women will again become all-powerful and will destroy them. Another reason for their fear of women who are demanding autonomy and equality is the idea that women will not be satisfied with equality — that they will want and demand dominance. Perhaps there is just a small amount of guilt intermingled with men's fear — after all, men were not content with equality, so why should women be?

Now, what about the women who label other nurses — and sometimes even themselves — witches?

There are many nurses, as I have said before, who are reluctant to work toward achieving a sense of autonomy and self-direction. They like the status quo. They never question, never disobey, never want to direct their own course. They use the myth of public submission-private power to hold onto their status-quo life. They seem to believe that the only way to exist is to continue to play the doctor-nurse game — to be the submissive, passive, subordinate hospital wife who is responsible for every aspect of housewifery that goes on in the hospital, whether that is pampering and coddling the hospital husband (i.e., the doctor) or taking care of the hospital children (the patients) so that they remain dependent and a little awed by this all-giving mother (the nurse).

So, to ask the question again, who gets called a witch in nursing?
Very simply, it is those nurses who have or are trying to get real
power — not mythical power — but power to control their own
lives and influence commensurate with their abilities in the external
world.

The women I'm talking about are not trying to attain omnipotence — they have no desire to dominate man and usurp his
place in his world. They are not power hungry, but they may be
envious of his unquestioned right to legitimate, political power.
They would rather be viewed as humans than as women. They
frequently demand equality, but I believe Janeway has a much
better idea when she speaks of reciprocity. She says, "A mutual
reciprocity of giving and receiving which is satisfying to both
partners seems to me the sustaining value of any relationship"
[6]. She happens to be talking about marriage, but as we have
already seen, there are many aspects in our relationships with
other health care professionals that are analogous to marriage, so
it seems to me that reciprocity is one of the few aspects that
could be seen in a positive light. Perhaps this is the way we can
transcend the fallacy of mythical female power and change attitudes and behaviors enough that there will be so few believers in
the myth that they cannot act to make it come true. What we
must do is to dispel the myth's plausibility, not try to prove it
false. "It matters not whether the myth is true or false, but
whether it is plausible" [worthy of being believed]. "As long as
the emotion invested in them can keep them plausible, they will
'work' well enough to get by, even though that isn't in fact very
well" [6].

How do or should nurses go about dispelling the plausibility
of mythical female power?

If we are going to use reciprocity to dispel this myth, it seems
apparent that nurses will need to increase the chances that mutually
satisfying relationships will be allowed to flourish. Certainly, it
takes some sense of willingness on the part of any two parties,
social systems or nations to establish mutually agreeable ground
on wh   tie build the relationsip. In other words, both men and
w   reg   ave to agree to some extent that what we might build
ou   new rocal interchange has some probability of being better
than what we have now. There will be times, no doubt, when

nurses will again be giving more for less, but that will level out as a true reciprocity begins to grow. In order to gain power, we sometimes have to give up power first. For instance, one of the reasons why some nurses are looked upon as witches is because of the ambiguity of whom they work for. Is it the patient, the doctor, the institution? I suspect that the answer will depend on whom you ask, but clearly, it will not be "for myself." For instance, at least one of the institution's expectations strains the relationship between nurses and doctors. The institution expects the nurse to be responsible for the physician's use of the institution's resources. After all, she is an employee of the institution and should, therefore, have some sense of loyalty to it in the matter of expenses incurred in keeping it functioning for patient care and as a place of employment! This expectation, of course, puts the nurse in one of her most uncomfortable roles. As Taylor [10] says, "The nurse cannot control the physician's use of these resources unless she challenges his medical decisions, and the nurse cannot openly challenge medical decisions" — particularly if she doesn't want to be looked upon as a deviant — a witch in nurse's clothing. She has several other choices, ranging from being a tale-bearer and informing on the physician, to making it difficult for the physician to find the supplies he needs, to evading the whole issue. Whichever choice she makes, she creates an unfavorable climate for developing reciprocity between herself and the physician, herself and the institution or herself and Nursing Service. One way out of this particular double bind is simply to institute a different organizational pattern in the Nursing Service unit of the hospital.

One that seems to work the best for the doctor-nurse-institution relationship is a unit manager system. Since there are a great many studies and reviews written about the system, I will not go into it here, but will simply say it frees the nurse so that she can be responsible for the management of patient care by introducing a unit manager to be responsible for the patient care *unit*. The unit manager is responsible for such tasks as seeing to it that the institution's resources are available so that both physicians and nurses can go about the business of curing and caring for patients In short, the nurse no longer has to "ride her broom" with to the business administration of the hospital. This is not idea or an original one — the Lysaught report proposed that "nurses be relieved of many of the non-nursing roles they have acquired over the years." The Commission then went on to recommend that "continued study be given to the use of technology, organizational practices, and specialized personnel (e.g., ward clerks and unit managers) that can release nurses from non-nursing functions while maintaining nursing control over the delivery of nursing care" [11].

Will nurses, given the opportunity, really then use their time in nursing functions? It is my opinion that the answer is both yes and no. Nurses are, first of all, human and have behaviors much like other human beings. So, some will become totally involved with patient care and some will fight to maintain their hard-earned territorial rights over the management of their domain. If this is what really happens, the next step may very well be to take a long, hard look at just what it is that makes those nurses so necessary to the provision of health care. I have no doubt that there are nurses who are good managers; however, I do not believe you can be a good nurse and a good manager simultaneously. Perhaps the administrative type should consider going into administration or management and give up the lip service about really wanting to care for patients.

In either case, the power base for nurses will change once we no longer have to be involved in the day-to-day management of the unit and become involved with the day-to-day management of patient care.

This change does not necessarily imply that nurses will become weaker or have less power. It can mean having much more power regarding decisions concerning patient care. In other words, the power base can be much more valid because the nurse will have to make decisions in an area where she knows what she is doing. Her credibility will be increased because it will be perceived by significant others on the team that she is an authority in nursing care.

It is the essence of power that the profession needs to cultivate in order to control our profession. We need to let the significant others of the health care team know in subtle and not so subtle ways that we have the knowledge, the ability and the power to make decisions about the nursing care we provide as part of that team.

Those nurses who do not have the knowledge and ability to be responsible and accountable for their nursing care will have to either seek other means of staying in the profession, such as further education, or stay in secondary positions on the team with no direct responsibilities for patient care. At any rate, they will have to reconcile themselves to the idea that our profession can no longer afford to protect and carry along those in it who do not want to become responsible and accountable for their nursing actions.

The 1970 census report indicates that 75 percent [8] of the workers in the medical-health care industry are women, and there are no predictions that it will change in the forseeable future. The political and economic power of the health care industry, however, still rests firmly in the hands of men who control it to their advantage and to our detriment. Without a political and economic power base, women in the field of health care will remain, as a group, powerless to control their own destiny. This powerlessness is not only a detriment to our profession but also a detriment to the patients we say we care for. According to the Lysaught report, research data indicate that quality nursing care can "(a) improve the actual treatment accorded the patient; (b) improve the economics connected with the delivery of health care; and (c) provide the personal reinforcement needed by the nurses themselves to deepen their commitment to the field" [11]. Quality nursing care is not likely to occur throughout the health care industry as long as nurses remain powerless to control their own practice. As long as employing agencies view nurses as secondary health care workers, a "warm body" that can follow doctor's orders, or a second-class manager for administration, and as long as they set pay scales that reflect these attitudes, nurses cannot attain or maintain a sense of their own worth or the worth of the work they do.

I realize that there are economists and health agency administrators as well as others who say that our present system is an efficient one. My question to them is the same as Pierce's: efficient for whom? She goes on to say that, "It must be remembered that efficiency only requires *someone* play the supportive role, belong to the maintenance class, devote their lives psychologically and physically to making sure that other people get done whatever they want done. As long as women as a class play supportive roles, they contribute to the efficiency of a power structure that keeps freedom of role choice for itself" [12]. As long as nurses as a group play supportive roles to other health care providers, they contribute to the efficiency of a power structure that keeps freedom of role choice, power and money for itself. A college-educated nurse invests about one-half the time in education that a doctor does and receives one-fifth the income [13]. According to Labor Bureau statistics [14], more than 50 percent of health care administrators have completed four years of college; however, the same statistics report that the annual median income for them is nearly $7,000 more than registered nurses with the same amount of education.

With this type of data is it any wonder that nurses drop out of the profession, particularly when much of the time we cannot provide the nursing care we have been educated to provide because we spend most of our time providing supportive care to others on the health care team!

But there is hope that the power structure can change. We can shift the balance of power in our direction by learning leadership skills and realizing that women in the health care industry outnumber men by a large margin. We need to develop leadership skills that include organizational effectiveness, goal-oriented behavior and creative risk-taking. Nurses must take the attitude that "the primary imperative for women who intend to assume a meaningful and decisive role in today's social change is to begin to perceive themselves as having an identity and personal integrity that has a strong a claim on being preserved intact as that of any other individual or group. This attitude will require women to develop an explicit sense of the value of their own concerns, and, at times to insist that they take precedence" [15].

Economics of Power

Along with changing attitudes toward careers for women outside the home and with legislation prohibiting employment discrimination based on sex, an increasingly service-oriented economy has brought both economic and social change to the status of women. Women, however, are still not in any appreciable number taking

210 advantage of the opportune climate that exists. According to one report from the Bureau of Labor Statistics, current figures on the employment of women are very similar to those of the past three decades. "The service industry ranked first in the employment of women" [8]. The same report states: "Many jobs in the service industry can be described as extensions of what women do as homemakers — teach children and young adults, nurse the sick, prepare food" [8]. So it seems that women usually get employment using the skills (or extension of those skills through education) they feel most comfortable with or in what they perceive as "feminine" jobs. Another contributing factor to women being in service industries is the readiness of employers to "allow" them to work part-time. Shift work or atypical hours are also attractive to women who have family responsibilities.

On the surface, it would seem that women, at last, have gained their place in the sun and have attained some control over their own destinies. And, to some degree, it is true. Nevertheless, for all our struggling, other statistics show we still have little or no economic power. Only one occupation out of the top ten best paid — physicians — includes even a small proportion of women — 9 percent. Half of all employed women earn less than $5,323 as compared to $8,966 for men; only 7 percent of women earn over $10,000, as compared to 40 percent of men; 10 percent of all families in the United States are headed by women; the median income of women with college degrees ($8,156) is little more than that of men with a grade school education ($7,535) [16].

Without power (money) to control our working lives, we are tied to an economic system that continues to exploit us just as it has in the past; even though we now have federal legislation that makes such exploitation a crime. And exploitation is not just limited to our day-to-day jobs. Consider, for instance, that it took Representative Bella Abzug of Manhattan two years to rally 74 sponsors for her bill to prevent sexist discrimination in extending credit. Even after two years, the bill had still not passed the House! Nor should we believe that once we reach retirement age we will receive equal consideration. Many groups, including feminists, recommend a complete overhaul of the Social Security system because of such discriminatory practices as this: "when both husband and wife work, the couple's benefits may be somewhat *smaller* than if the total family earnings were the same but only the husband worked" [17]. Do single women fare any better? Not much. Social Security benefits are based on what has been earned during the time of employment. "Low wages during employment means inadequate social security on retirement, thereby condemning millions of retired working women to a life of poverty" [16]. Private pensions are not much help either. Most working women (those in service industry, for instance) may not be eligible for pension plans because of the kinds of jobs they have or because they work part-time. It soon becomes evident when one reviews these data that our passivity can lead us into and keep us in a state of poverty. "Given their fear of success, their under-estimation of their own endeavors, society's negative — or, at least, ambivalent — attitude toward success and power in women, and, of course, their limited opportunities, it is not surprising that the ultimate success positions in this country have never been occupied by women" [17].

There are a few rays of hope amidst all the gloom. In 1973, individual women owned 18 percent [16] of total shares of stock of public corporations; a nationwide survey in 1973 determined that 4 percent of the applicants for executive positions were women [17]. This was an 800 percent increase over any other year. All government contractors or subcontractors with at least fifty employees and contracts worth $10,000 or more are required by law (since late 1968) to have affirmative action programs clearly specifying hiring and promotion policies toward women. This, of course, includes virtually every large company, research organization and educational institution. "In fact, women's groups have now filed charges against almost every university and college receiving federal funds and against most major corporations" [17].

One fact remains clear though — the relationship between levels of income and numbers employed in any occupational category is a negative one: as the proportion of workers who are female increases, the relative income for women in that occupation decreases. This illustrative of what I call a "double bind." The more we gain in terms of fields of occupation, the more we lose in terms of income.

Are nurses doing any better than other women? Not to any

great degree. It is true that hospitals have been gradually catching up with long overdue improvements in wages and working conditions for both professionals and nonprofessionals. The prevalent view that payroll costs are the primary reason for increases in hospital costs has not been true for a number of years, however. "From 1960 to 1967, despite a 17 percent rise in personnel per one hundred patients, total expenses per patient day advanced more rapidly than payroll per patient day, 68 percent against 62 percent" [18]. "As late as 1946, the Department of Labor documented the fact that nurses in the United States worked longer hours, did more night and shift work, received less overtime pay, had fewer fringe benefits, and were paid lower salaries than most workers in industry or in comparable occupational groups" [19]. The net effect of this, plus the fact that large numbers of nonprofessionals are joining the ranks of hospital workers, has been to perpetuate what the Lysaught report quotes Anderson on: "In the past a large part of the servers — professional and non-professional — in the health services system were paid less than prevailing wages because of the non-profit and eleemosynary nature of health care and the dedication presumed to be expressed by the workers in being willing to care for the sick and disabled" [11]. Long hours, low pay, poor working conditions and lack of identity and recognition have forced many nurses to drop out. They no longer practice or have much interest in returning to active practice. "The system of health care is frequently the cause for nurses leaving nursing, and it is this very system that must be modified if we are to progress toward needed changes in nursing" [11]. The National Advisory Commission on Health Manpower had much the same thing to report: "There is a crisis in American health care . . . *The crisis, however, is not simply one of numbers . . . unless we improve the system* through which health care is provided, care will continue to become less satisfactory, even though there are massive increases in costs and numbers of personnel" [20].

"The hospital system of health care has exploited the nursing profession, used its cheap productivity, and ignored its cravings for dignity and respect" reports Trucia Kushner in *Ms.* magazine [21]. Certainly, I have to agree with the sentiments expressed because they are true; however, nurses are the ones who have allowed this to continue long after there was any need for it to. Florence Nightingale may well be given the credit for establishing nursing as we know it — including low pay, long hours and subservience to men — however, this is the twentieth century now and other professions have managed to leave their pasts in the past. Nursing needs to do the same.

The Women's Movement and the health care crisis is a combination of events that can pull nursing out of its nineteenth-century attitudes into the "now" world. Nurses are beginning to see themselves as the obvious answer to huge gaps in this country's health care. Efforts by nurses to make nursing a high-status profession will not only improve their economic power base but will ultimately improve patient care as well. In the final analysis, nurses must become aware of their self-importance, or, as stated earlier, women (and nurses) must develop an explicit sense of the value of their own concerns, and, at times, insist that they take precedence. Nurses with this stand will pose a tremendous threat not only to other members of the health care team, but also to other nurses who are not interested or involved in changing the status, power or economic base of nursing. There is power and a certain amount of political clout in most of the new Nurse Practice Acts — New York's, for example; yet few nurses seem to recognize it or are able to use it effectively. "To be responsible and accountable" (and get paid accordingly) "for the delivery of nursing, we must have the authority to act and to do what is necessary to deliver this essential service" [22]. The new Nurse Practice Acts, for the most part, give us that authority to act. Our own sense of the value of our concerns will convince the public that we have a service of great value to deliver.

References

1. Morgan, Robin. Rights of Passage. *Ms.,* Vol. 4, No. 3, September 1975, p. 98.
2. Ashley, JoAnn. This I Believe about Power in Nursing. *Nursing Outlook,* Vol. 21, No. 10, October 1973.
3. Gamson, William. *Power and Discontent.* Homewood, Ill.: The Dorsey Press, 1968.
4. Schattschneider, E. E. *The Semi-Sovereign People.* New York: Holt, Rinehart and Winston, 1960.

214   5. Gamson, William. Violence and Political Power — The Meek Don't Make It. *Psychology Today,* Vol. 8, No. 2, July 1974.

6. Janeway, Elizabeth. *Man's World, Woman's Place: A Study in Social Mythology.* New York: Dell, 1971.

7. Parsons, Talcott. *The Social System.* New York: The Free Press, 1951.

8. Waldman, Elizabeth, and McEaddy, Beverly. Where Women Work — An Analysis by Industry and Occupation. *Monthly Labor Review,* U.S. Department of Labor, Bureau of Labor Statistics, May 1974.

9. Nin, Anais. *Diary, 1931–34.* New York: The Swallow Press, Harcourt, Brace and World, 1966.

10. Taylor, Carol. *In Horizontal Orbit.* New York: Holt, Rinehart and Winston, 1970.

11. Lysaught, Jerome P. *An Abstract for Action.* New York: McGraw-Hill — Blakiston, 1970.

12. Pierce, Christine. Natural Law Language and Women. In *Woman in Sexist Society: Studies in Power and Powerlessness,* Gornick, Vivian, and Moran, Barbara (Eds.). New York: Basic Books, 1971.

13. McBride, Angela. Leadership: Problems and Possibilities in Nursing. *American Journal of Nursing,* Vol. 72, No. 8, August 1972.

14. Sommers, Dixie. Occupational Rankings for Men and Women by Earnings. *Monthly Labor Review,* U.S. Department of Labor, Bureau of Labor Statistics, August 1974.

15. Adams, Margaret. The Compassion Trap. In *Woman in Sexist Society: Studies in Power and Powerlessness,* Gornick, Vivian, and Moran, Barbara (Eds.). New York: Basic Books, 1971.

16. Jongeward, Dorothy, and Scott, Dru. *Affirmative Action for Women.* Reading, Mass.: Addison-Wesley, 1973.

17. Doyle, Nancy. Woman's Changing Place: A Look at Sexism. *Public Affairs Pamphlet No. 9,* June 1974.

18. Somers, Herman. Economic Issues in Health Services. In *Contemporary Economic Issues,* Chamberlain, Neil W. (Ed.). Homewood, Ill.: Richard D. Irwin, 1969.

19. Bullough, V. L., and Bullough, B. *The Emergence of Modern Nursing,* 2d. ed. New York: Macmillan, 1969.

20. *National Advisory Commission on Health Manpower,* Vol. 1. Washington, D.C.: U.S. Government Printing Office, 1966.

21. Kushner, Trucia. The Nursing Profession — Condition: Critical. *Ms.,* Vol. 2, No. 2, August 1973.

22. Fagin, Claire M. Nurses' Rights. *American Journal of Nursing,* Vol. 75, No. 1, January 1975, p. 271.

8 Changing

Marlene Grissum

In an important sense this world of ours is a new world, in which the unity of knowledge, the nature of human communities, the order of society, the order of ideas, the very notions of society and culture have changed and will not return to what they have been in the past [1].

Robert Oppenheimer

for Tomorrow

Change is frightening to most people. Eric Hoffer, in *The Ordeal of Change,* states that "we can't really be prepared for that which is wholly new" [2]. We must make adjustments, and this creates a crisis in self-esteem. We perceive that a change is a test of ourselves and we have to prove outselves. Of course, this takes a measure of self-confidence, not only to face the change but to allow ourselves to be tested in the new situation. Hoffer also says that change is one of the agencies that release human energy. What is nursing doing with the human energy we have released now that nursing is in a state of change?

We in nursing have been using a great deal of our released energy trying to understand the process of change itself and trying to understand each other. Change has caused some confusion because there has also been a change in our professional language. Our vocabulary now includes: accountability, accessibility, responsibility, expanded role, extended role, rights, economic and general welfare, mobility, militancy; the list could go on and on. Do we really have a unified, clear understanding of our new vocabulary? Do these words mean the same to me as they do to you? Is our concept of nursing as a changing profession and a change agent within our society understood and shared by others? "Change agent refers to the helper, the person or group who is attempting to effect change" [3].

The evidence indicates that the general public still believes that nurses are extensions of physicians with no ability to think, no responsibilities and, certainly, no accountability to anyone other than the physician. This concept of nursing and nurses is perpetuated by the media (for a more in-depth analysis, see Chap. 6), the public and many nurses. But there is also a "new breed" of nurses who do not see themselves as stereotypes and will not allow the media, the public and other nurses to go unchallenged when that stereotypic picture of them is presented. The nurse with this new attitude will be a change agent within our profession. Stanley Peterfruend has pointed out what he calls the "new breed" [4] in the American work force, and it is certainly present in the nursing work force today.

Attitudes toward Change

A rise of individualism or, put another way, the drive for personal identity and recognition, is one of the characteristics of the new breed. Peterfruend asserts that workers in industry are "hungry for personal recognition; they want to work in an environment in which they don't have to bury their identity" [4]. This need is noticeable in nursing as well, and it illustrates why nurses are proclaiming, loud and clear, that nursing is not an extension of medicine, that nursing is a profession separate but equal with any other profession. Great numbers of nurses are no longer satisfied with being nameless faces that never question; that always respond to someone else's idea of appropriate behavior; that always respond to a stimulus from others but rarely initiate a stimulus to themselves or others.

True, the unsettling nature of any change creates anxiety in those involved. And, certainly, that is true in the nursing profession today. Side by side with the "new breed" of nurses are the "old breed," who are satisfied with the status quo. The old breed are not interested in personal identity and recognition. They do not feel that endless paper work, telephoning, secretarial tasks and assistance to the physician are meaningless work. They are not even aware that they are oppressed, both as women and as nurses. They receive their rewards by pleasing others whom they see as superior. Their definition of meaningful work is not the same as that of the new breed nurses. It does not include the concepts of autonomy, self-actualization, commitment and self-realization — as they relate to the profession of nursing. Their attitudes, as demonstrated through their behaviors, indicate that they believe their role is to continue the passivity and dependence that is inherent in the age-old ideas of femininity. These same nurses help to perpetuate the idea that the traits of compassion, tenderness and understanding are limited to the female. The new breed nurses must be aware that because of the old breed nurses, the old system is perpetuated (either consciously or unconsciously), salaries are kept down, women are kept down and the nursing profession is kept in its second-class status. Change can and is occurring around them, but because of their anxiety level about change and their unwillingness to expend their energy on it, our efforts as change agents are more costly in time, money and energy.

Up to now, nurses who are change agents have not really been conscious of going about instituting change on a *planned* basis. If we are to initiate change on the large scale I believe will be necessary, however, we must begin to look at change in a planned, orderly, rational manner so that what is accomplished is what *we, the change agents,* want accomplished. Is there a question of ethics if we manipulate others so that they accept our values, attitudes and beliefs? Some behavioral scientists seem to think there is. They believe that it is a responsibility of change agents to clarify their own values and the temptations that exist to use their influence to narrow and foreclose rather than to widen and release the free choices available. "We know that we are no longer choosing wisely when we choose within the framework of assumed and unexamined traditions of belief and practice. We are literally legislating the future for ourselves and for others as we choose and act upon our choices. *Since our value orientations are at least partial determinants of our choices, responsibility requires that we become clear about and responsible for our actual as well as our professed ideal values as they function or fail to function in*

the choices we make as change agents" [5] [italics mine].
Even if we do not hold the belief, as many behavioral scientists
do, that "any manipulation of the behavior of others constitutes a violation of their essential humanity" [5], we do
have to be aware that effective behavior change always involves some degree of manipulation. Of course, there are many
situations in which all of us would consider manipulating others'
behavior as ethical, such as human rights, education or some
aspects of patient care.

Change and Conflict
There are a variety of theories concerning planned change,
ranging from the psychological point of view as expressed by
Erickson through the social communication aspects as seen by
Bauer to the new tradition of organizational leadership by
McGregor [5]. These all have one theme in common, and that
is conflict, because some form of conflict is an inherent part
of behavioral change. Therefore, persons who desire to be
change agents should be aware that conflict will occur when
change is advocated or instituted. In our American society,
conflict or disagreement regarding basic values or the roles
assigned to each group tends to be regarded as destructive
[6]. We are socialized to believe that adjustment, not conflict, is better. This socialization process, including our need
to be liked, is inculcated to the extent that the individual
feels guilty about expressing unorthodox or unpopular views.
Our survival chances, as a nation or as individuals, to some
degree depend on our abilities to meet change and resolve
the conflicts it causes in some reasonably positive fashion.
Constructive and creative conflict resolution will continue to
be of primary concern to professions that are interested in
helping people who are involved in change.
Needless to say, that involves everyone to the extent that
they are involved in the social milieu of our society. At
times the rate of change is incomprehensible to us. Some
people greet each new change with joy and enthusiasm, while
others resist change every inch of the way. But whether we
like it or not, whether we are joyful participants or outraged

spectators, change is accelerating. The rapidity of change and the results in human behavior have been called a new disease, or *future shock*. Toffler claims that future shock is a time phenomenon, a product of a greatly accelerated rate of change in society [7]. Time is used as a yardstick to measure change because there is no absolute way to measure it. So, we say the rate of change is the number of events that occur within a fixed time period. With that frame of reference, it becomes very easy to understand our own uneasy feelings about how fast change occurs. In past centuries, one could live out a lifetime without experiencing any real change in society. But within this century, change has accelerated to such proportions that the overwhelming majority of all material goods we use in daily life today have been developed in our time [7]. And, of course, change is not limited to the material goods we use, but also to knowledge, situations and the psychological responses of humans. For instance, Toffler claims there is a parallel between the accelerative curve of book publication and the rate at which humans discover new knowledge. And Philip Siekevitz, a biochemist, claims that "what has been learned in the last three decades about the nature of living beings dwarfs in extent of knowledge any comparable period of scientific discovery in the history of mankind" [7]. Furthermore, there is nothing to indicate that the rate is decreasing.

In other words, change at an ever-accelerating speed is a part of our world. We need to become more and more aware of that as well as aware of how one goes about adapting to it and to the conflicts that are an inherent part of it. Knowledge about conflict and conflict resolution is an extremely important aspect of our daily lives whether we are men, women or children. We all deal with a variety of stresses in a variety of social situations where the ability to resolve conflict is necessary for our physical or psychological survival. Constructive conflict resolution leads to more open lines of communications, new interests, insights and curiosities about human behavior. "Often, as a positive consequence of conflict, new pathways of communication and new group relationships may occur. Sometimes, conflicts force one to re-examine one's stereotypic images, perceptions, and attitudes towards other groups, and to change

222 or restructure these perceptions toward more accurate ones"
[8]. In contrast, there are also some destructive aspects of
conflict and its resolution. Perceptions about conflict that are
destructive include the myth that conflict is bad. There are some
aspects of conflict that can color the perception of what it is all
about. For instance, if conflict is strong enough, it can be harmful
to individuals and groups. It may be overwhelming to those who
have no mechanisms for resolving it. Anxiety and fear may be
intensified in conflict situations so that the person wishes to
withdraw, becomes apathetic, feels immobilized and generally
insecure. Certainly, other destructive consequences can occur
when conflict is received in overwhelming doses to the person
or the group. Most social scientists, however, agree that there
are more positive aspects to the phenomenon than negative
ones.

Several definitions and theories have come into use concerning
conflict and its resolution. For instance, Bennis et al., in *The
Planning of Change,* list among others: (1) conflict as a result
of different and incompatible goals for change held by various
parties within the same situation; (2) conflict that is a result of
the struggles over the allocation of commonly prized goods —
whether money, material goods, power or prestige and status;
(3) conflict that stems from perceived threat to their very identity
as persons or groups between and among parties to the conflict[9].

According to Mack and Snyder, conflicts may be viewed as
micro (small) or macro (large); realistic (incompatibility of values
and interests); nonrealistic (need for tension relief, hostility
deflection or ignorance and error) [8]. Conflict can also be
categorized in a variety of other ways such as: institutional,
noninstitutional, direct, indirect, cultural, sociological, psychological, economic, religious, or sexual. In other words, the
list is as diverse as humans are. Rogers [10], however, believes
that a collaborative relationship turns out to be the most important aspect of conflict resolution, especially if the change
endeavors to be healthful and growth-producing.

It is not the intent in this chapter to investigate change and the
ensuing conflict on a global or theoretical level. Rather, my purpose
is to examine it in the context of the health care industry and,
more specifically, how it relates to nurses.

Today, nurses and the rest of the health care professionals are
faced with change that is as rapid in our professions as it is in
the larger society. Future shock is as much a part of the health
care industry as it is of the space science industry. Furthermore,
it is often perceived as a threat by nurses and others in our sphere.
For instance, the entire concept of intensive care units, including
the tools, equipment, knowledge and personnel to staff them,
has become a "normal" part of an acute care hospital within the
past ten to twelve years. Up to that time, acutely or critically
sick patients were a part of the regular unit of a hospital floor
and were cared for by the staff. This necessitated a more diversified
staff as well as a larger one. In many instances, families paid for
private-duty nurses to stay with loved ones who were critically
ill. The changes wrought by the onset of intensive care units involved everyone working in the hospital as well as patients and
their families. There was really no need to have sophisticated
equipment in the ICU if there was no laboratory to make needed
tests; hence, the laboratory staff felt the change. There was less
need for private-duty nurses because the nurses working in the
intensive care units took care of critically ill patients, and only
those. They were, in one sense, providing private nursing care
for the patients in the ICUs; hence, private-duty nurses felt the
change. Nurses who were employed in hospitals at the time of the
first ICUs and were asked to be on the staff or volunteered for
places on the staff of the ICUs soon realized that they needed
extra training in order to be able to use the complicated equipment; also, their transfer to the ICUs left gaps in the nursing staff
on the regular units; hence, nursing felt the change. Certainly,
administration had to be involved, because the increased need
for space, equipment and staff had to be dealt with in the budget;
hence, administration felt the change. Patients and their families
were intimately involved and felt the threat very personally.
Patients were more frightened by the equipment, noise and awe-
someness of an ICU than they were of the rest of the hospital.
Families also were extremely frightened of the whole concept.
The idea that a member of their family was confined to a special
room with special people working in it and that they could not be
with the patient was enough to make them even more anxious

224 and concerned for their loved one. And there was no one to talk with about the patient as there had been when there was a private-duty nurse. Moreover, they had little or no knowledge concerning why certain procedures were being carried out. Hence, patients and families all felt the change. The list could go on and on through every department in the hospital. Just this one change in the care of acutely ill patients reverberated through the entire staff of the hospital and into the community. The resulting conflicts had to be resolved on each level before ICUs could become functional to any great degree. It seems apparent that interdepartmental and intradepartmental collaboration resolved most of the conflicts that ensued as this one change became a part of the health care industry. Change continues to take place in this important area of health care (as it does in others), and the resulting conflicts over new and more advanced equipment continued to be dealt with in all areas of the hospital.

One issue involving advanced technology that has not been resolved is the definition of death. As our ability to sustain life becomes more and more technologically advanced, the conflict becomes more intense. This conflict will not be as easy to resolve as the ones surrounding the staffing of ICUs because it involves some very fundamental issues, such as: What is life? And what is death? The answers necessary to its resolution will be extremely difficult for those involved in the search. It has been noted, however, that when a conflict reaches crisis proportions, human beings *must* resolve the crisis within a short period. Undoubtedly, this issue will involve some collaboration between those parties involved.

With this very superficial description of one very small change that has occurred in the health care industry, it is not difficult to realize that change is an inherent part of our lives and that there are other areas that are changing. Perhaps the changes will not be viewed as quite as dramatic as those involving ICUs; however, many of them can create as much conflict. For instance, the whole concept of expanding the skills and the roles of nurses is another area of change that is fraught with conflict. Our attempts at resolution continue and certainly will involve many different methods of conflict resolution. Five or six years ago, when the idea of expanded roles for nurses first came into full bloom, a great

felt highly threatened by it. Many nurses felt threatened because
they feared they could not cope with an expanded role but would
be forced into one. Others felt threatened because they perceived
the change as doing doctoring, and they wanted no part of it.
Still others were anxious to begin — they felt there was very little
about the concept that was really new. In fact, they perceived it
as an opportunity to be able to provide *real* nursing care, an
opportunity to get back into contact with the patient; but they
felt threatened by the idea that they would not be *allowed* to do it.
Physicians also saw it in a diversity of ways. Some were extremely
threatened because they viewed it as an infringement upon their
control of the patient. Others saw it as a threat because it would
"dilute" the medical care patients received. Apparently some even
saw it as a threat to their masculinity to have their territory
invaded by women, especially women who were not even doctors.
Others saw it as a beautiful opportunity to use nurses as physician
assistants and were not threatened at all until the nurses' professional organization took a firm stand on one discipline stealing
staff from another discipline in order to lighten their own work
load. The conflict still rages, and a firm one-answer resolution to
it has not been found. Strides forward have been made in many
areas however, and as expanded roles for nurses come into full
fruition we can anticipate changes in other areas.

Those areas of health care where the conflict seems to have
been resolved most successfully for all concerned include pediatrics,
family health care, maternal health care and geriatrics. More and
more nurses and physicians are learning to collaborate on a professional peer basis. The resultant opportunity to provide health
care rather than just illness care is extremely rewarding for the
providers as well as for the patients. According to Leininger,
other areas where we can anticipate change, and therefore conflict,
include: (1) ways to provide health care delivery in an economical
and humanistic manner; (2) ways to provide financial support for
professional education; (3) changes in practice and use of new
ideas in education and services; (4) ways to deal with collective
bargaining in educational and service settings; (5) ways to insulate
practitioners from the prevailing economic job-management focus
when it neglects the professional growth and patient welfare aspects;

(6) ways of retaining standards without neglecting public accountability; (7) ways to heighten productivity, responsibility and social
accountability of professional health care workers [8].

When one considers the three basic types of conflict stated
earlier plus the areas of conflict or potential conflict listed above,
one realizes that the means of initiating change are as important
as the ends or the conflict resolution. The primary question is:
what methods, strategies, processes and models related to change,
conflict and conflict resolution could provide new insight and
alternative choices to health care professionals?

Confrontation

Carl Rogers' *collaborative relationship* theory [10] is one answer.
To use it, the change agent must be willing and skilled at using
confrontation. We must seek, according to this theory, limited
and realistic bases of collaboration and build upon them, without
denying different interests and orientations. It is claimed that
collaboration is an achievement, not a gift. We are warned that
change agents who anticipate that collaborative ways of working
will occur without mutual confrontation, effort and learning have
a limited understanding of either collaboration or conflict [10].
This theory corresponds to Leininger's method called *open and
direct confrontation* [8]. The parties involved confront each
other regarding the issues that are producing the conflict. They
must remain open, direct and willing to collaborate in an effort
to come to terms with controversial issues. For the most part,
nurses are at a disadvantage using this method because, as women,
we have not been taught the fine art of confrontation. Confrontation takes aggression, self-confidence and knowledge of
the issues as well as the ability to communicate in a direct, open
manner. It is part of our socialization as women to be passive,
dependent, nonaggressive and to communicate indirectly. It
becomes readily apparent that the skill needed to use confrontation well is something nurses will have to learn. Nursing leaders
are encouraging and recommending the use of open and direct
confrontation as an effective means to resolve major issues within
our profession as well as with other professionals. In our society,
however, we have very few women, and even fewer nurses, who

can use it effectively right now. In fact, Sandra Bem found, in studies she conducted on 1,500 undergraduates at Stanford University, that women who consider themselves feminine find it difficult or impossible to behave in an aggressive manner [11]. Their ingrained sense of femininity (being dependent, passive and nondirect) restricted them to behaving in the typical feminine way. They would even lose money in order to avoid behavior that they perceived as masculine, i.e., assertive, aggressive or independent. When put into a situation where they had to perform trivial masculine tasks, such as hammering nails into a board, they described themselves as feeling less attractive and likeable, more nervous and peculiar, less feminine, and they did not enjoy the experience [11]. Professional nursing is fortunate to have several leaders who are skilled in confrontation, but we need to increase the number tremendously if nursing is to have an equal voice in resolving conflict and instituting changes in our health care system. Mutual respect, trust and goal achievement can, and often are, the end results of confrontation when it is used skillfully by both parties. Frustration, anger and hostility can result when confrontation is used by one group against another group which is not skilled. The end results will be an increase in the conflicts between the two groups. It seems apparent that the incentive for women to use it effectively is there; what is needed is education in its use.

Power and Change

Power is usually gained or lost in the resolution of most conflict, but what many nurses do not seem to realize is that social action (change) depends on power in much the same way as physical activity depends on energy. Power is not necessarily a bad thing, despite the apparent fear it generates in a great many women. A successful change agent tries to utilize power that is based on and guided by rationality, knowledge and collaboration to achieve change and resolve conflict.

Richard Walton has proposed two strategies for change based on power tactics involving maximum use of potential power to achieve the change desired. There are two major steps in using power strategy to gain the goal. "First, in order to establish a

228 basis for negotiation with the other and improve the probable outcome for itself, the group must build its power vis-a-vis the other. Group A can increase its relative power by making Group B more dependent upon it and by decreasing its own (A's) dependence upon B. Often change is sought by groups with a relative power disadvantage" [12]. Sometimes, in order to command attention and establish an exchange basis, one group must threaten the other group with harm, loss, inconvenience or embarrassment. Leininger calls this the organized mediator-arbitration method, or the industrial model [8]. She asserts that power is a factor, and that a strong opposing power base can overwhelm a weaker one. Thus, groups must assess their power and, if it is weak, find means to strengthen it in order to be successful in negotiations. Obviously, Americans are familiar with this method and recognize it as the one most likely to be used by both labor and management to settle most contract negotiations. Nurses will become more familiar with the intricacies of negotiations using this method as more and more nurses form bargaining units within their places of employment. To participate, one must understand the special terms used, such as arbitrator, negotiator and manager, as well as what each person's role is in the process. Strikes, marches and speeches are techniques that are sometimes used to bring issues to the attention of the public and the involved groups.

A second step in the power strategy or industrial model is required in order for one group to maximize use of its power or potential power. That step involves changing the rival group's perceptions of the strength of the other group and how committed they are to achieving their goals. For instance, the leader of group A attempts to overstate his group's needs or preferences for achievement of their goals. He may also depreciate the importance of group B's goals to group B's leader. Needless to say, these attempts require skilled leadership abilities. There can be no ambiguity or uncertainty on the leader's part. The communication must be manipulated so that it appears to B that A is totally committed to a course of action and that B does not have time to get his group together to commit themselves to a different set of actions. Illustration of this tactic in use can be found in the foreign policy decisions by our country. Walton cites the Cuban missile crisis, the Berlin crisis and the war in Vietnam.

It is important for the group making the threat to carry it through if the situation requires it. For instance, the United States did indeed increase the bombing of Vietnam. Many times, of course, the threat does not have to be carried out, such as in the case of the Cuban missile crisis. The opposing side removed the missiles from Cuba without added power being exerted by the United States.

In a more peaceful vein, one could observe the same process occurring with the striking nurses in San Francisco in June 1974. At the beginning of their negotiations, they used the threat that they would strike if necessary in order to gain their goals. When it became evident that the opposing groups were not willing to negotiate a contract with the nurses' goals included, the nurses carried out their threat. By doing so, they increased their power base, gained their objectives and won a strong position in the health care industry for their area.

There is a certain element of risk involved as each group attempts to assess the strength of the other group regarding the threats. Each leader must take a gamble on how far the other side really means to go. Each group must be cohesive and supportive of their leader in order for the other group to recognize the power and strength of their opposing group. Frequently, the strategy is played out across the bargaining table and the threats and counter-threats do not have to be used. Many more conflicts are negotiated peacefully than are negotiated through strikes and shut-outs.

There is another strategy of change, advocated by Walton, that seems applicable to nursing; it is based on changing attitudes of the opposing group. Attitude change strategy [12] depends on increasing the level of attraction and trust between groups. Instead of maximizing the group's potential power, attitude change strategy recommends minimizing the perceived differences between the groups. Communications to the rival group stress peace rather than violence. Considerable emphasis is placed on the mutual dependence of the two groups as well as equal status for their respective members. Attempts to achieve a high degree of empathy with respect to motives, expectations and attitudes between the groups are an integral part of the strategy. This strategy is analogous to Leininger's friendly persuasion and interpersonal skills model [8]. Actually, it is the most common method used

230 to resolve conflict in our society. It is used daily by all of us as we go about the process of living our daily lives. For instance, most marital conflicts, child-parent conflicts, employee-employee conflicts and employer-employee conflicts are resolved using persuasion, subtle inducement and personal appeals. Even if the conflict cannot be resolved using this method, it is likely to be tried first before we progress to other methods.

There are other methods of conflict resolution that can be used by change agents. The more skillful and knowledgeable we become in the different methods, the more apt we are to recognize which one is most applicable and when it is appropriate to use it. We also need to understand them in order to recognize which ones the rival group is using against us. These range from the supernatural to revolution [8]. Some of them would be difficult or inappropriate for nurses to use in resolving the conflicts of our professional growth. There is, however, one other method mentioned by Leininger that seems to have a great deal of validity for nurses. She calls this method the "mutual alliance or common pact of several different groups" [8]. This method has not been widely used in the western world, but it does have applicability for women who are involved in the health care field. It is based on open discussion between several divergent groups that are also involved in the same conflict. Through a series of meetings, these divergent groups discuss and negotiate their different interests as well as their common goals. Mutual interests and respect for one another are usually the outcomes of such discussion. The process is dynamic, and the best resolution agreement is brought about through the group process. Through the dynamics of group process, several leaders emerge that represent the different groups. They must be highly perceptive, respected and skilled group leaders. The principle by which the group leaders function is to allow divergent views and interests to expand and contract while at the same time holding the whole group together.

This method of conflict resolution should be thoroughly investigated by all women in the health care industry, primarily because even though we have much diversity between our interests, we also have a great deal in common, and particularly because we have only second-class status in an industry controlled by men but run by women. This method would accommodate our diverse interests while allowing us to be a democratic, cohesive group. In other words, each group is allowed to remain individualistic (nurses and social workers do not have to agree on everything), but each group is involved with and has the support of the others in resolving conflicts we all share. Although there are a myriad of different interests involved, women in the health care profession have several areas of common interests. The paucity of women in leadership roles within the health care industry is one major area that should concern all women involved. The duplication of effort in attracting women with leadership qualities to the health care field is another area — not to mention the time, money and effort that each group expends separately in attracting drop-outs back into their profession. Certainly, the situation of women professionals being powerless and subordinate could be eliminated by joining together to negotiate changes with the more powerful, male-controlled areas of the industry. The group thus formed could also become a clearinghouse for the divergent groups to be aware of what methods other groups have used in the past to gain power, create change and resolve conflict for us or against us. It becomes quite obvious that many of these strategies have been used against nursing in the past. For instance, by substituting the word *medicine* for group A and the word *nursing* for group B, it is not difficult to see how the power strategy has been used against nursing.

This analogy corroborates what Ashley asserts: "History shows that physicians very early recognized their own increasing dependency upon nurses. As nursing power became manifest, physicians came to believe that nurses had to be intellectually and socially controlled" [13]. Such manifestations of power in nursing and reactions to this power led to the development of the doctor-nurse game form of communication between us. According to Ashley, this form of communication, when it first began, was an effort by medicine to control nursing power and minimize nursing's influence [13]. As scientific knowledge increased, medicine's practice base increased. At the same time, physicians developed stricter controls over who could practice as well as who defined what the practice of medicine was. Because they set very firm guidelines and stringent definitions of practice, they were able to decrease their dependency upon nursing, while at the same time

232 increasing nursing's dependency on them for orders, prescriptions and regimens of care. Even though this process actually started in the fourteenth century during the witch burnings [14], it culminated around the beginning of the twentieth century in this country. "In 1910, the recovery of patients, more often than not was the result of the nurse's activities and not those of the physician" [14]. The skilled nursing care that a surgical patient received saved more lives by preventing infection than the surgery itself saved. In fact, without a knowledgeable nurse, most patients did not survive. Physicians freely referred to nurses as their colleagues and professional allies; their dependency on nursing was evident in their actions and words. It is interesting to note that nurses at that time had not yet become attached to hospitals as their source of patients and income. It could be said with some validity that as nursing's dependency on hospitals increased, physicians' dependency on nurses decreased. A great number of nurses continued to work as independent practitioners who made their financial arrangements directly with the patient up to the time of the Depression. So, even though the physician may have been instrumental in obtaining the nurse for the patient, he had little or nothing to say about the nursing care she provided.

When we consider attitude-change strategy, it becomes apparent that this too has been used to decrease further the power of nursing. There are hospital administrators, physicians and nurses who frequently try to minimize the perceived differences between the groups' goals and between characteristics of members of the groups. One statement that is heard frequently is: "After all, we're all on the same side — we are all trying to take care of the patient." Another area of emphasis is the degree of mutual dependence. This is frequently discussed as the need for teamwork. Such statements as: "Team effort is what it really takes to care for the patient, and we are all part of the team." In reality, astute nurses know that teamwork can result in good patient care and that it probably should be the optimum we strive for. Nevertheless, in actual practice, many times the team functions only as long as it benefits the other members getting their functions completed. And it only functions as long as the physician remains the team leader. In other words, the team functions as long as *cure* takes precedence over *care*. (*Cure* and *care* concepts are

covered more fully in another chapter, but are based on *cure* being
a function physicians perform and *care* being a function nurses
perform.)

Fortunately for patients and providers, the concept of teamwork
is beginning to be really understood by more and more health
care providers. In many areas it has become the modus operandi
in meeting patients' needs.

There are tensions involved in dealing with any of the strategies
of change and conflict resolution. What choice a professional group
makes depends upon the creative and collective efforts of the group
in choosing the most effective and available resource. Very few
situations are so clear-cut that one would know without question
which strategy would best apply. But the theorists do give us some
clues in order to make more knowledgeable decisions. "Mixed
or dual strategies can be pursued more readily by an organization
than by a person, and more readily by a movement than by an
organization" [9]. In other words, we need to be able to ascertain
whether the conflict can best be dealt with at an individual, organizational or movement level and proceed accordingly.

The whole idea of equality for women is a movement, and
change that results in conflict will have to be viewed in terms of
its globalness. Certainly, it seems that combining one or more
strategies is the better way if the conflict involves all women in the
health care industry. It is not difficult to imagine the force we
could exert if all women in health care banded together. Using
the mutual alliance method plus the power strategy method to
attain mutually beneficial goals such as control over our own
areas of practice, we could become a major force in changing the
health care industry. Change agents in nursing need to take a
long-range view so that overall goals are defined as well as short-
term ones. In doing so, we may be able to see when it is advantageous
to use power strategy and when another strategy would be more
apt to accomplish our goals. We should be cognizant of the fact
that substantial gains by means of the power or industrial strategy
are more likely to be realized if an improvement in attitude is first
established. One area where this idea is of extreme importance is
our own profession. If change agents can effect an attitudinal
change in nurses concerning power and its use, we can then be
better assured that we have cohesive support to attempt similar

234 changes in relation to other groups. The point stressed by Walton is that attitude change may result in some lessening of conflict and some increase in trust and confidence [12].

The reverse of this viewpoint is that, in some instances, it will be profitable for us to use power strategy first. This almost always results in a temporary setback in interpersonal relations with the other group. In the long run, however, the results may be better relations. If, by using power strategies first, we demonstrate our commitment and our self-respect, we may engender respect from the other group. This occurs because if "a group must be treated differently (more equal), there is a tendency to regard them differently (more equal) in order to make one's beliefs and attitudes congruent with one's behavior" [12]. One example of power strategies being used profitably is in bargaining. Commitment, promises, threats and threat fulfillment are usually part of the negotiations that take place between an employer and employees. Sometimes the only avenue open to the group is its capacity to harm the opposing group. Frequently, if not always, this is the operant cause of a strike. The striking group has no other means of asserting its power.

That there may be dilemmas involved in choosing the best tactics should not be overlooked; but dilemmas should not completely paralyze us so that no action takes place. Nursing education usually provides for developing insights and skills in the strategy of "attitude change," or the "friendly persuasion" method. Nurses, therefore, may find they will be more comfortable and knowledgeable in using this, which in no way implies that we should use this strategy to the exclusion of all others. What it does imply is that nurses will be less fearful in trying to change attitudes than they will be in trying to exert power. Because there is so much confusion concerning conflict and its resolution and because nurses have not used strategies to any great extent, it is vitally important that we be aware of the various methods and when to use them. We cannot hope to be a part of the resolution if we do not understand the processes involved and our own feelings, fears and ambivalences concerning conflict.

Individual change is probably more painful and traumatic than organizational change for most of us. So the first step in coming to grips with our personal feelings regarding change and its ensuing conflict is to become involved with what is happening in our profession. There are a variety of ways to do this, including participating in our professional organization, continuing education, consciousness-raising groups or other ways such as reading. Whatever combination is chosen, it should open avenues to the acceptance of new ideas concerning our womanhood and nursing. Osta Underwood recommends that we be willing to give up the comfort of predictability and become aware of the unconscious programming that shapes individual, corporate and cultural lives. She also recommends that we know the "tools" that are available against discrimination and how to use them to initiate change [15].

In recent years, many laws have been enacted that deal with discrimination in employment. In fact, there have been so many different laws, executive orders and guidelines that both employees and employers have difficulty in keeping up to date. For instance, the Fair Labor Standards Act of 1938 was amended in 1961, 1966 and 1972. All three changes expanded the act and made it a stronger weapon for employed women. The changes primarily brought more people coverage under the minimum wage and overtime provisions of the act. Many of these, such as retail employees, were women. With the changes of 1966, the act extended coverage to include employees of state and local hospitals, schools and colleges. Again, this extended coverage to a large number of women. There is really no way to estimate how this act has increased the power of women to be more autonomous. It is likely, however, that there are a great many women employed today who do not know of its existence, do not know what it can or has done for them and do not know whether their employer has to comply with its provisions. Consequently, they are not aware that they can use this act, along with many others, to make sure changes are instituted in their places of employment to achieve better working conditions for themselves and other women. I am not implying that all employers are criminals who are deliberately breaking the law, but it is possible — because of misunderstanding the changes, or ignorance of them or malice aforethought — for employers to be paying less than the minimum wage.

The same is true of the other laws enacted to protect workers such as the Equal Pay Act of 1963. Women should be aware that this is the only provision in any law which is confined exclusively to sex-based discrimination. It requires that men and women performing equivalent work must receive equal pay. When first enacted, it did not include employees in executive, administrative or professional capacities. In 1972, it was expanded to provide coverage for an estimated 15 million executive, administrative and professional employees. Four to five million of these were women. Again, women need to be aware that they can use this law to help them bring about changes in their place of employment.

Title VII of the Civil Rights Act of 1964 is probably women's most potent tool, since it applies to discrimination in all terms and conditions of employment. It forbids an employer to discriminate between men and women in hiring, discharge and compensation and in terms, conditions or privileges of employment. Since Title VII became law, there has been at least one suit filed against every major university in the country. For instance, "the American Nurses' Association filed charges against the nation's largest university pension underwriter March 1973 for discrimination on the basis of sex. The complaints, the first to be lodged by a national organization on the issue of discrimination in retirement benefits, were filed on behalf of three women professors who are ANA members" [16].

There are other laws and guidelines that are of interest to women, but these illustrate the point that women can institute changes in their employment situations and that the power strategy of change can be used by being aware of the laws that exist.

On a work-related basis, we need to know the organization well, especially key people in powerful positions. Presentation of the issues in such a way that the key person will support your stance is a necessary leadership characteristic for women in general and especially for nurses. Certainly, one of the primary requirements in instituting change is to study the issues well. Having adequate data to corroborate your charges and being knowledgeable about both sides of the issue is to your advantage. A change agent needs to be conscious of the myths that abound in our society about women. Some of these are such a "normal" part of socialization that we tend not to question their validity. Well-founded research that is up to date will help dispel the myths. Change agents also need to collect data that will counteract the use of myths by those in key positions, particularly when they use them as excuses for continuing actions that are discriminatory in nature. One such myth used against nurses is that they are extensions of medicine; therefore, there is no need to define nursing as a separate profession. Another is that hospitals will be responsible for the actions of nurses in cases where malpractice suits are brought against nurses and the hospital.

We also need to be aware that in most large organizations there are several systems that seem to exert negative pressure on women who aspire to succeed. One such is a "visibility system" [17] that controls the upward mobility of those in the organization. Visibility is one of the primary elements of upward mobility. "One must be seen before one is recognized" [17]. Without recognition there is little possibility of climbing the ladder of success. In most instances, women's visibility is based on sex, not achievement, and of course in nursing the problem is compounded by the fact that it is a woman's profession. Nurses need to identify the visibility system that operates in their place of employment and start using methods of change that will alter it to the degree that achievement is more visible than the sex of the achiever. Right now nurses are more apt to be viewed by the administration, the public and other members of the health care industry as a mass; nurses are perceived as *nurses* rather than individuals. In the eyes of those who control our health care organizations, there is no differentiation between the nurse who is an LPN and the nurse who is a Ph.D. In order to change the concepts held by others regarding who is a nurse, we need to use attitudinal change along with friendly persuasion to get the message to those in control. Needless to say, when more nurses become articulate activists involved in changing the system, those with whom we negotiate will be more likely to recognize nurses for their achievements rather than their visibility or lack of it.

Women's jobs frequently reflect the status assigned to them by our society, and nursing is no exception. Another system working against women is the property value system [17], which is based on the concept that woman's work is of less value than man's work, even when they are doing the same thing. When less dollar value is placed on work, less power will be ascribed to it. The organization, whether that is health care or government, does not necessarily create the attitude by putting a dollar value on jobs. They are merely exploiting an advantageous situation. It is imperative that women become aware that we are being exploited and take action to rectify it. "We must become aware and willing to identify, confront, and make personal and/or professional adjustments necessary to change" [17]. A thorough knowledge of the laws available to assist us in making the necessary changes is, of course, one of the ways to take action to rectify the exploitation of women. Other means include those change strategies reviewed in this chapter. Learning how to be a skillful change agent; to communicate, confront, negotiate, legislate, compromise and revolt are all necessary in the life of a change agent.

Women have always held a very precarious position in the labor market. Like many of the minorities, we have always been expendable, to be called or rejected in relation to fluctuations in production, sales, patient, client or student load. At present, employers are actively seeking nurses in most parts of the country. But that does not necessarily imply that discrimination is less likely to occur, or that changes are not needed. It does imply that nurses probably have more of an opportunity to initiate changes within the health care system now than at any time since the early nineteen-hundreds. In the past, nursing has not used the advantages that are inherent in a supply-and-demand situation. Surely, we have passed the stage in our growth and development as a profession where we see bargaining as nonprofessional or as unethical. We can change the balance of power in our favor by using one of the change strategies in negotiations to receive more pay, better working conditions, control over our own practice, and implementation of programs designed to increase the quality of patient care we deliver. We can use the laws available to us to make sure that no woman is discriminated against because she is a woman. Furthermore, it can be accomplished on a national, state and local level so that *all* nurses benefit, not just a few who have the courage to confront the system with well-planned strategies.

In order for our potential power to become real, nurses must unite so that common leaders can be found and given a mandate to negotiate for the changes we need. With the right leaders, and by using strategies designed to implement changes, nursing will be a more nearly autonomous profession with more open power to help patients through our ability to get decisions and plans implemented. The biggest fallacy among the health professionals, according to Leininger, is the philosophy of sharply dividing our conflicts. With such a strong dichotomy, we limit a wide range of possibilities for all those involved. Our effort to see everything in an either/or fashion keeps us separated from other professionals with equally dichotomized views. We need to be able to accommodate and tolerate differences of opinion and other viewpoints. Even more importantly, particularly for women in the health professions, we need to endeavor to understand such differences and work toward some degree of cohesion. Almost all of us realize that compromise is a daily event. In order to survive, we have to adapt, to give and take, in any conflict situation. As health care professionals, however, with the health of others involved, we must not compromise too easily or too readily. We must be willing and able to make sound assessments; to negotiate with reason and from positions of strength, social justice and respect. To yield our professional values, ethics or major goals too easily may have serious consequences for ourselves and others [8].

In the past, some antagonism toward change has been generated among the elements that make up the health professions. At times, also, the people involved have failed to see a need for change. The times and the conditions, however, are *now* significantly different than ever before. For one thing, it is a common feeling among nurses and others that the nursing profession must change in order to ensure minimal requirements for future patient care. For another, the American public is now much more involved in the process of decision-making regarding health care for this nation. As national health insurance becomes more likely, public participation will increase. The public and the professionals are becoming more and more aware that industrial, social, electronic and biomedical changes have been occurring for some time in our present system. These changing patterns broaden health care opportunities, but they also create more problems. Given the best of all possible worlds, the American public would choose to go back to receiving personalized care from the family doctor. At the same time, they expect the latest technological advances to be at their disposal if they need them. Their expectations of nurses are much the same.

240 They want the "lady with the lamp" to provide personalized care in traditional and acceptable ways, but also to be knowledgeable enough to be able to monitor any equipment they may need. "Thus, the central problem for all health professionals becomes how to control and implement change — how to incorporate today's advances with the still-useful practices of yesterday" [8].

Somewhere between the myths of the past and the mists of the future, nursing stands with the potential to be the key to maintaining a humane, individualistic concern for people and their health problems. Our efforts as change agents must be directed toward the ultimate ideal of better health care for our society. To be able to accomplish that goal, we must be willing and able to attack our educational system, the roles of women in general and nurses in particular and the hierarchy of the present system that continues to perpetuate its own inadequacies.

The public will also have to be involved in the changes that must be instituted. One reason our present system is such an abysmal failure is because the population has increased enormously — while maintaining their desire for "private" health care at a reasonable price. Our society needs to start looking for innovative ways to receive health care that indeed help them maintain their health. The whole idea of health maintenance is another area in which the public needs to become involved. In the past, the public depended on health care providers to *make* them well rather than to *keep* them well. In order for our present system to sustain itself at all, the public must begin to bear some of the responsibility for health maintenance. We simply must get rid of the myth that there is a pill for all ills. The emphasis must be placed on *staying* healthy rather than *seeking help only when ill*. Right now, the high cost of being sick is exceeded only by the high cost of staying healthy. The whole health care system is geared toward curing illness. For instance, up until a very few years ago, health insurance rarely covered health maintenance care. In other words, the insurance was collectible only if the person was ill and hospitalized. Finally, insurance companies are becoming aware that it is probably less expensive in the long run to keep patients out of the hospital if at all possible.

In the past, doctors and nurses were educated to be disease-oriented, and they still are in many areas of the country. Surely, physicians need to be skilled in diagnosing and treating the myriad of illnesses that beset humans. Somewhere in the process, however, they have lost interest in *keeping* people well. Hence, this is *one* of the reasons why other health care professionals need to expand their skills. I am not implying that all physicians are disease-oriented, but what I am saying is that we need more people who are health-oriented, including the public. I am also saying that more people need to be educated toward disease prevention and health maintenance. Whether those people are doctors or nurses is really not the question — our society needs to be educated to how they can be a part of the team to maintain their own health. For too long, the average American has operated under the assumption that if he became ill, the doctor would cure him. In the meantime, he did not have to *do* anything to stay healthy. In other words, the entire responsibility for his health or lack of it rested in the hands of the physician. There was a sort of magical belief system working in the American public that empowered the doctor with the necessary ingredients to make them well again. Fortunately, many people in our society have now given up their beliefs in magic. Many more are becoming aware daily that, in the long run, their state of health or illness depends on their own ability to be responsible people. The public has finally reached the stage where they can allow the physician to come down off his pedestal — to be a human rather than a demigod. It can only be hoped that this trend will grow.

The concepts of change and conflict are stimulating, exciting and growth-producing. Both change and its conflict can help us to see new or different ways of thinking and doing. Somewhere in the maze of change, conflict and conflict resolution lie answers to the perplexing problems that are besetting the health care industry today.

For instance, what is the best way to resolve the conflict between what the consumer wants and needs and what the health care industry can provide? Is the answer in realistically but mutually held goals and objectives provided through discussion between the two groups, i.e., friendly persuasion? Will the answer lie in some form of national health insurance, i.e., power strategy? Is there some way to use open and direct confrontation methods to resolve the conflict? Perhaps some entirely new method of conflict resolution will provide the answers. Probably it will be a combination of all these as well as others that finally does solve the conflict as we know it today. This does not mean that conflict will no longer be there. Change is a fluid, dynamic process that will, we hope, always be a part of our lives, because without it we would not exist. All living things experience change and all experience some form of conflict with that change. The resolution of conflict is what makes life such a beautiful challenge and gives us the energy and stamina to try again tomorrow.

References

1. Oppenheimer, Robert. Introduction. In *The Planning of Change*, 2d ed., Bennis, Warren, Benne, Kenneth, and Chin, Robert (Eds.). New York: Holt, Rinehart and Winston, 1969, p. 1.
2. Hoffer, Eric. *The Ordeal of Change.* New York: Harper & Row, 1963.
3. Oppenheimer, op. cit., p. 5.
4. Peterfruend, Stanley. The Challenge of the "New Breed." *Nursing Digest,* Vol. 2, No. 7, September 1974. Condensed and reprinted from *Michigan Business Review,* January 1974.
5. Kelman, Herbert. Manipulation of Human Behavior: An Ethical Dilemma for the Social Scientist. In *The Planning of Change*, 2d ed., Bennis, Warren, Benne, Kenneth, and Chin, Robert (Eds.). New York: Holt, Rinehart and Winston, 1969.
6. Presthus, Robert. *The Organizational Society.* New York: Random House, 1962.
7. Toffler, Alvin. *Future Shock.* New York: Bantam, 1970.
8. Leininger, Madeleine. Conflict and Conflict Resolutions: Theories and Processes Relevant to the Health Professions. *The American Nurse,* Vol. 6, No. 12, December 1974.
9. Bennis, Warren, Benne, Kenneth, and Chin, Robert. Introduction to Chap. 4, Collaboration and Conflict. In *The Planning of Change,* 2d ed. New York: Holt, Rinehart and Winston, 1969.
10. Rogers, Carl. The Characteristics of a Helping Relationship. Introduction to Chap. 4, Collaboration and Conflict. In *The Planning of Change,* 2d ed. New York: Holt, Rinehart and Winston, 1969.
11. Bem, Sandra. Androgyny vs. the Tight Little Lines of Fluffy Women and Chesty Men. *Psychology Today,* Vol. 9, No. 4, September 1975.
12. Walton, Richard. Two Strategies of Social Change and Their Dilemmas. Introduction to Chap. 4, Collaboration and Conflict. In *The Planning of Change,* 2d ed., Bennis, Warren, Benne, Kenneth, and Chin, Robert (Eds.). New York: Holt, Rinehart and Winston, 1969.
13. Ashley, JoAnn. This I Believe about Power in Nursing. *Nursing Outlook,* Vol. 21, No. 10, October 1973.

14. Ehrenreich, Barbara, and English, Deirdre. *Witches, Midwives and Nurses.* Old Westbury, N.Y.: The Feminist Press, 1973.
15. Underwood, Osta. Legislation and Litigation: Impacts on Working Women. In *Affirmative Action for Women,* Jongeward, Dorothy, and Scott, Dru (Eds.). Reading, Mass.: Addison-Wesley, 1973.
16. *The American Nurse,* Vol. 5, No. 4, April 1973.
17. Daddio, Saundra. Oh! The Obstacles to Women in Management. In *Affirmative Action for Women,* Jongeward, Dorothy, and Scott, Dru (Eds.). Reading, Mass.: Addison-Wesley, 1973.

9 On Becoming a Risk-Taker

Marlene Grissum

*The fence around woman's place is
more apparent to the people who live
inside it than to those outside in
man's world [1].*
Elizabeth Janeway

and a Role-Breaker

Part of the feminine ideal, the ability to please, is usually looked upon as a virtue, especially by men. It is an attribute commonly expected of women and other subordinates by the powerful [1]. Also, it will probably be the first *female* virtue that women who are to become risk-takers will have to discard. Central to the idea of getting rid of it is the idea that "the powerful do not please. It is the subordinate who must do so" [1]. This idea — that power negates the necessity for pleasing — not only keeps women in subordination, but it is also confusing as well. It brings more fragmentation into the already fragmented world of womanhood. "One cannot dedicate oneself wholly to doing, and being, what is good if one must at the same time consider how to please, for the two sets of standards may well conflict" [1]. The woman who sets out to be a risk-taker has a formidable task before her; she needs to use her energies and intelligence to achieve being fulfilled in her role as well as to bring about the changes that are her goals. Women have been socialized into rigid, inflexible roles that have limited them in goal-directed activity to that which is

246 pleasing to their *superiors.* All women should be aware that any woman who acts persistently in an unpleasing way is not just committing a blunder; she is deliberately moving counter to what society says is the traditionally acceptable role for woman. She is becoming a "role-breaker" [1]: a deviant whose behavior provokes hostility and fear.

To play any role, one must use the expressive behaviors that society has assigned to that role in order for the role to be understandable to others. In the past, there has also been another requirement connected with women's roles. A woman's behavior was supposed to indicate that it was by the grace of her superiors that she acted at all — hence, pleasing had top priority. According to Janeway, shame is "the penalty for not pleasing" [1]. No one in our society enjoys feelings of shame, but women are doubly fearful of it because avoiding public shame is part of our socialization as women. Confronting shame "requires an ability to risk . . . disappointment, frustration and ridicule" [2]. It also involves a sense of vulnerability. High-risk-takers are open, much the same way that a child is open, to those around them. Their openness leads to their being extremely vulnerable, in both the positive and negative connotations of vulnerability.

The intent of our risk-taking and role-breaking is to break the stereotyped molds that have held us in a nonfunctional state since the last wave of feminism. The secondary position of women is the mold that has caused us all to be cast in the same role: that of helpmate, nurturer, *beloved imbecile.* To break that mold and assume an equal but different stance alongside the opposite sex is the great task before all feminists, which, of course, includes feminist nurses. The role of women and the role of nurses are so inexplicably woven together that there is really little need to designate which one is being discussed. When role-breakers make strides forward as women, role-breakers will make strides forward as nurses. Women who are role-breakers and who also happen to be nurses will be able to use the gains made in both their social and work roles. It has been said that the women's liberation movement is a state of mind, and so too is the idea of being a risk-taker and role-breaker. Nurses who take risks and break the stereotypic roles they have in the work situation cannot then expect to be submissive, coy, passive women in their larger social world. The two concepts are not congruent. Twenty years ago, de Beauvoir claimed that the majority of workers were exploited. Even though woman's condition at that time was better than it had been, the world still belonged to men and still retained the form they had given it. Women who are role-breakers and risk-takers will change the world's form so that it is more human-oriented than man-oriented. Now, as then, workers are exploited, and the exploitation of women workers has changed very little. Even though new laws enacted in the past five years make this illegal, it still continues.

Nowhere is this more obvious than in the profession of nursing, where the very characteristics that keep us down as women are needed so badly to provide quality health care. Feelings of compassion, tenderness and nurturance that have traditionally been described as feminine are the very ones that our professional education and experience tell us are the essence of good nursing care. They are also the very ones that men use against us, however, when we attempt to assert ourselves and become controllers of our own destiny. Because we have been socialized to accept pleasing our superiors as *normal,* we can be publicly shamed when we make demands and agitate to change the system. We frequently get caught in the bind of feeling guilty that our demands will, in some way, be harmful for patients since these demands are ego-centered. The *giving* component of nurturance, fed by our fear of shame, blocks our attempts to better our own lot, even when we know that by increasing our own stature we can provide better care for patients. This situation is analogous to what de Beauvoir described as the object and prey [3]. The conflict that results as we try to clear up the ambivalence we feel concerning our own needs and how we feel about them in relation to our patients is one aspect of being emancipated that is difficult to resolve. We are torn between the desire to assert ourselves and our desire to remain self-effacing.

One way we resolve the conflict is by being easily reconciled to a moderate amount of success. Woman enters her profession (nursing, for instance) only half prepared because she really believes it is not her primary commitment; then she only superficially invests her time and energy in her work and simultaneously wonders why she has no power, no respect and no fulfillment. Women like having a job and knowing that they are capable of handling it properly; but they are not passionately concerned with the *content* of their tasks. Role-breakers are not satisfied with being capable. We need role-breakers in nursing who also want to be accountable, responsible and autonomous. "Role breakers should be prepared to find themselves under attack, regarded as unattractive and frightening, running into hostility" [1]. We, as role-breakers, need to be willing to take that risk. Understanding *why* hostility and rejection are likely to occur can often help us as we strive for the changes our profession needs. Because role-breakers destroy ascribed patterns of behavior, significant others no longer know how to respond. Fearful that *their* response will be inappropriate — will cause them public shame — they respond with anger and hostility.

Knowing that hostility will occur and why it occurs can give us an edge by allowing us to prepare ourselves for it. We need not wait for the attack; we can take the attack to those who express anger. Being on the offensive rather than the defensive is a politically astute maneuver that has been used against women many times. By turning the tables, we gain two advantages. We have our offensive attack prepared, and we bring the element of surprise with us. Heretofore, women have not been well versed in the tactics of offense. We more often reacted after the fact — we responded to a stimulus; we did not initiate the stimulus. Confronting those in the health care system who react with anger toward nurses who are breaking stereotypes and demanding nurses' rights can be an exhilarating experience, particularly to those who are skilled in the art of confrontation. Role-breakers must be knowledgeable regarding the issues, articulate in expressing them and skilled in using confrontation and negotiation to gain their ends — a leadership role in the health care of this country, power to control our own profession and autonomy for our individual practitioners. "This means nursing must be willing to take a stand on issues and people. We must be willing to commit ourselves publicly to what we believe about nursing, health and society. We must take the lead — we must take the risk" [4].

Political action and involvement are certainly parts of any role-breaker's role. According to Max Weber, "Politics is the striving for power or striving to influence the distribution of power" [4].

When nursing is fragmented, has no leadership, is busy running from one group to another to define and defend itself, nursing's power is weakened and it makes nurses easy prey for the opposition to continue to exploit them as nurses and as women. "The political power of nursing can be defined by its value as a profession to society, its numbers (over one million strong), its ability to stand up and speak out for what it believes with one uniform voice. Naturally all of these power areas need to be expanded and channeled by capable and unafraid nursing leaders" [4]. The expansion and channeling are the tasks of the role-breakers and risk-takers in our profession who either are or will be our nursing leaders. Twenty years ago, when women were being told that they were indeed the *Second Sex,* de Beauvoir declared that "only those women who have a political faith, who take militant action in the unions, who have confidence in their future, can give ethical meaning to thankless daily labor" [3]. Nursing apparently paid little or no attention to what de Beauvoir had to say then, but surely we can see now that we need those same kinds of characteristics today to give meaning to our "thankless daily labor." We can no longer afford to let the larger health care society set our goals, dictate our behavior, control our power — particularly when we consider that by virtue of our numbers, we are the larger health care society!

In order to reverse this process we need to identify our nursing leaders. We need to recognize the knowledgeable, competent, articulate practitioners, educators, researchers, wherever they are — who can be the spokespersons for and unifiers of nursing. When we identify them, we will find they are the risk-takers, the role-breakers who dared to be different. They are the nurses who will demand their right to practice nursing as defined by our profession rather than as it is defined by other members of the health care team. Role-breakers (hence our leaders) will be found in every health care setting, doing all levels of nursing care. They will be the nurses who are not well liked by administration, not respected by some of their peers, feared and distrusted by physicians but loved and respected by fellow role-breakers for their courage, intelligence and future-oriented outlook. They will be the knowledgeable, competent, articulate practitioners, educators and researchers who can infuse new life into a profession that is becoming root-bound and archaic. They will create feelings of hostility, anger, awe, respect, love, admiration — in other words, emotional tensions that will release energy to set our profession into a leadership position in the health care field. After our profession is once again moving and is the dynamic, viable profession it once was, we need to "use all of the ways available to us to make nursing visible as a positive force in the health care field" [4]. We then need to use our articulate, knowledgeable leaders — our role-breakers — to stress our positive strengths, contributions and accomplishments to the public, other members of the health care team, legislators and nurses. This whole strategy, as explained in Chapter 8, can best be accomplished by one united organization that speaks for all nurses.

Needless to say, with over a million nurses available, not all can be leaders or role-breakers on a national level. That does not negate the fact that we need to have the skills, the courage, the commitment and the ambition to follow their example. Role-breakers are needed on every level and in every aspect of nursing. We need to incorporate the characteristics of a role-breaker so deeply into ourselves that wherever we are and whatever we are doing, we *are* role-breakers and risk-takers. We need to learn how to talk instead of listen, question instead of answer, contradict instead of acquiesce, demand instead of comply. We must deny the idea of the "unconditional supremacy of man" [3]. There is no supremacy — nor can we ever allow it to exist. The world, the health care industry and the people who work in it have too much to do to expend their energies on valueless enterprises such as maintaining the myth of male supremacy.

Everyone's life is a succession of challenges and self-affirmations because everyone has some degree of self-limitation — some lack of assurance that engenders it. For the most part men, because of their socialization process, see the challenges as opportunities to reaffirm their positive image of self. Women, for the most part, see the challenges as dangers to what small strides they have made. It is an opportunity to reaffirm their negative image of self. They are more likely to seek to make good in prescribed ways rather than aim toward some goal that they have formulated for themselves. This is the type of behavior that role-breakers can no longer allow to exist. They are willing to take the risk — to aim for the goal — to

reaffirm the positiveness of self. Does that make them masculine?
No, it makes them more likely to succeed — more confident —
more self-assured — more responsible for setting goals and reaching
them. There is no time left to consider whether something is
masculine or *feminine*. What is important is whether or not it
is *human* — in the most beautiful sense of that word. "The continuing concern of any society must be to avoid freezing behavior
into roles that were appropriate to past situations but have now
lost so much of their utility that they invite misunderstanding"
[1]. Role-breakers make us very cognizant of one thing: "It is
possible to move away from one stereotype with impunity, if there
is shelter near another" [1].

In the past, whenever women became role-breakers and departed
from one female role, they took up another one. Nursing is illustrative of this point. It became acceptable for women to become
nurses and to work outside the home because nursing was viewed
as women's work. They departed the role of mother, housekeeper,
house manager at home for another role very similar in nature.
Freezing the role of nurse at that level is one concern that this
society has not dealt with. That role was perhaps appropriate at
the time, and some facets of it still are. The role, however, has lost
so much of its utility that it does indeed invite misunderstanding.
It has hardened into discomfort. We must indicate clearly to the
public and to our profession that that role is no longer appropriate.
The social situation has changed, and our behavior will also change
to meet new aspects of our role as nurse. "When women step out
of their role they very often upset the people they are working
with. That makes for trouble, and trouble costs money. At this
point a balance appears. Is it cheaper to keep women working in
traditional and accepted ways only to lose the potential talent
and energy they might bring to new jobs? Or will there be a big
enough payoff to make the trial worthwhile?" [1]. Janeway
declares this is an empirical question, but perhaps it is not, where
nursing is concerned. When one considers that the payoff may
well be better health care for our society, the trial certainly seems
worthwhile. To keep nurses working in traditional and accepted
ways means to keep them from using a broad base of scientific
knowledge based on research — a process that affords nurses an
opportunity to use that scientific knowledge — and patients from

receiving the benefits. It may well be economical from the point of view that traditional and accepted jobs for nurses are pitifully low-salaried, but it doesn't appear to be economical to society as a whole when one considers the dearth of good health care available to that society.

The issue really is not what is economical; nor is it that some physicians are now delegating some of their tasks and responsibilities to nurses. The issue is that health care services are changing, and health care providers need to adapt to meet those changing needs. The central focus of nursing is care, comfort, guidance and assisting individuals to cope with health problems that range from being healthy to being ill.

There are nurses who will claim that we who accept these delegated responsibilities from physicians are no longer nurses but physicians' assistants — that we have sold out — become the "Aunt Janes" of the health care system. These same nurses think nothing of taking a patient's blood pressure (once the sole responsibility of physicians) or giving patients medications ordered by the physicians. (There was a time when the physician carried the medication in his bag and he alone gave it to the patient. The nurse was not even allowed to know what it was he gave.) We can no longer afford such rigidity in either profession. We need to be able to "distinguish nursing *practice* from the practice of nurses, which includes ministration of medical acts delegated by the physician to the nurse" [5].

Role-breakers and risk-takers will be found assuming the responsibilities delegated to them not because they want to be pseudo-physicians, but because they have the skills to assume those responsibilities which will obviously help them in providing health care. Lambertson's analysis of two-dimensional nursing practice, one structured and defined, the other unstructured and ambiguous, is helpful in identifying where to find role-breakers and risk-takers [5].

Nursing leaders will be found in the unstructured and ambiguous patterns of practice. Lambertson's definition of this pattern of practice is exactly my definition of what a role-breaking nurse will be found doing: "1) Those tasks or functions that involve potential hazards or risk of safety (physical and emotional) or therapeutic outcome. 2) Those tasks or functions that are perceived to be required in an uncontrolled situation. 3) Those tasks or functions that involve alternatives of choice in predicting or projecting courses of action. 4) Those tasks or functions that are unstructured and require reordering of knowledge in their design and implementation" [5].

It can be assumed that more and more nurses will function as primary health care providers, with their practice directed toward assisting people to maintain their health, rather than either supporting or contributing to the physician's practice of diagnosis and treatment of acute illnesses. This seems an obvious division of labor between the two professions, especially in view of the alleged shortages of nurses and physicians. If the assumption is correct, nurses will have to be willing and able to function in unstructured and ambiguous situations. A nurse will also have to stop seeing herself as "an underling, one who cannot make decisions, cannot take risks, should not promote one's attributes for economic gain, cannot take command unless given a specific title and specific job description" [6].

All-encompassing generalizations about nurses and physicians must be swept away to be replaced by definitions of nursing and doctoring that are based on the individual skills, knowledge and judgment exhibited by the persons involved and that are required for safe, efficient health care for people in our society.

As more and more physicians and nurses are educated together and learn to appreciate the different but equally important skills each brings to the health care setting, we can anticipate more collaboration between the two professions. But before this can occur on any large scale, role-breakers must be willing to take the risks and blaze the trail for those who will follow. "Women must convert their 'love' for and reliance on strength and skill in others to a love for all manner of strength and skill in themselves. Women must be able to go directly to the heart of physical, technological and intellectual reality as they presumably go to the 'heart' of emotional reality. This requires discipline, courage, confidence, anger, the ability to act, and an overwhelming sense of joy and urgency" [7].

As women in general and nurses in particular learn to go directly to the heart of physical, technological and intellectual reality, they will become more assured that the health care of this society

254 depends upon their ability to *assume* the leadership role. (It won't come any other way.) Chesler states that: "It is clear that women who are feminists must gradually and ultimately *dominate* public social institutions in order to insure that they are not used against women" [7]. The public social institution of health care has traditionally been used against women — both as patients and as providers. In the not too distant past, and perhaps even now, women have been incarcerated in mental hospitals for being role-breakers — for refusing to play the game of happy housewife, for daring to question male supremacy. We now have the potential economic and political power to see that such injustices are forever banned in our society. We no longer have to depend on fathers, husbands and brothers to bring home the money to support us. In almost all instances we have the opportunity and the ability to support ourselves, even though we usually are paid less for our labor. What we, as women and as nurses, need now are enough risk-takers among us to assure ourselves of an equal if not dominant place in our social institutions. We need women who are willing to take the risk of being called crazy — who are willing to bear hostility — willing to be different — in order to reach a place outside "woman's place." It is a sad commentary on our place in society that right now hospitals, communities, government and organized medicine exert more influence on nursing and its future than our own profession can or does [8]. Role-breakers and risk-takers must assume positions that will allow them to exert influence to correct such injustices to women and nurses.

Nancy Keller seems to imply in her article on the nurse's role that in order to *save* nursing we will have to give up the ideas that nursing is a profession and that nurses are professionals. She advocates going back to technical nursing because it offers "an exact, unambiguous sort of opportunity to professionalize the work instead of the worker" [8]. She totally discredits nurses who are assuming some of the skills that up to now have been the sole prerogative of physicians by making the false and absurd assumption that nurses cannot possibly benefit from learning or using them — that we will only be assisting the physicians and the profession of medicine. "As we move to assist the physician more officially and in greater numbers, then they are free to press for a large stake in the reorganization of health care delivery" [8].

She completely ignores the idea that much of the power of any profession is mandated to it by the public it serves. If nurses who are willing to take the risks involved fill the gaps that are so apparent in our health care system, we may very likely find ourselves being mandated much of the power that society has heretofore reserved only for the providers (physicians) of the health-illness care they have received.

Dr. Catherine Norris takes the position that "direct access to one's patient or client is mandatory for a profession" [9]. She goes on to assert that many of the problems inherent in the inability of nursing to assert itself as a profession and of nurses to act autonomously could be resolved by obtaining and maintaining direct access to the patient. What better place than at the point where patients enter into the health care system? "Direct access to patients, as demonstrated in experimental models, requires commitment. The nurse must be committed to function professionally in meeting health needs. This means that she must lay claim to the parts of health care which *she defines* as nursing, and that *she must take full responsibility for her own functioning and her own decisions.* Short of this, there is little point in direct access, in autonomy, and in professional education for practice" [italics mine] [9].

This, then, could very well provide nursing with all the necessary tools for controlling our own professional lives as well as our lives as women in this society. By obtaining and maintaining our direct access to patients, as well as the patient to us, we have the potential to provide better patient care, to develop more effective means of delivering care and to gain the power necessary to control our own destiny. Surely that is incentive enough for many of us to become role-breakers and risk-takers. The hostility and anger we will have directed toward us seem little enough to bear if we can know that we are instrumental in changing the pattern and focus of our whole health care system as well as changing the pattern and focus of the practice of nursing. The one trap that nurses must make certain they do not fall into is in assuming "the autocratic exclusiveness of medicine where the physician tells everyone what to do" [9].

Is the field of primary health care of interest to nurses? Are they willing to assume the responsibility and accountability necessary to acquire a position as a role-breaker? Some data certainly seem to indicate a positive answer for both questions. Research done by McCormick and Crawford shows that "the desirability of the primary care role for nurses was good or excellent by 88.5 per cent of respondents; only 6 per cent thought it undesirable. Sixty-five per cent of the respondents indicated personal interest in a primary care nursing career; eighty-five per cent of the respondents thought it would improve the professional image of nursing" [10].

This research seems to indicate that there are more than a few nurses in our society who are willing to assume the risks involved in becoming role-breakers. They are ready and anxious to try to crumble the images of traditional nursing and build a new image based on their own and others' ideas about what nursing has to offer society in regaining and maintaining a healthy state. What we need is a unifying force that will set us on the course of becoming responsible for our own destiny. That unifying force could very well be our professional organization utilizing its growing political clout to get us out of the doldrums and into the action. It may also be the women's movement that pulls us into the real world and out of the unreal past by forcing us to see that nurses are their own worst enemies. It is interesting to note that McCormick and Crawford's data also show that "Many who stated they themselves would not consider this career mentioned marital and child rearing responsibilities as precluding employment" [10]. That kind of attitude will be used against us just as it has been in the past to keep us in our secondary positions. The women's movement (which is really not a movement but a state of mind) may be the force that will show nurses that their commitment to *their* profession is as important as their husband's commitment to his. It may be the force that gives them insight into the idea that parenting should not be the exclusive domain of mothers, but a shared responsibility of both parents, if not of others who are significant in their lives. Perhaps they may gain enough self-assurance and self-esteem to realize that they can be role-breakers in all areas of their lives; that they do not have to merely dream about how nice it would be if they could only do something like nursing.

Social scientists, among others, have been scrutinizing the changing role of women rather carefully within the past decade, particularly in regard to changing fertility patterns. Data from a 1970 reveal that most women do not hold beliefs that are totally "traditional patriarchal" nor totally "egalitarian feminist" in nature. Even though there seems to be a mixture of beliefs and outlooks, the data do reveal some rather discouraging statistics. For instances, "almost 80 per cent of the 6,740 ever-married women under age 45 said that 'it is much better for everyone involved if the man is the achiever outside the home and the woman takes care of the home and family'" [11]. One wonders how many nonpracticing nurses were among the 6,740 respondents. Another revealing piece of information gathered from this survey is that barely a majority of those responding believed that women should be considered for the best-paying and most responsible jobs. The author believes this suggests that "the female public may still tolerate considerable differences in the treatment of women and men workers" [11]. There was continuing strong support for the segregation of basic roles by sex, but "nearly half the women interviewed felt a woman should not let children stand in the way of a career if she wants it" [11]. One of the controls that restrict women from choosing a career while their children are small, however, is the social pressure against mothers who "neglect their children." This, of course, is a social pressure that is most likely to be exerted against white, middle-class women. Poor women, both black and white, are expected to work in order to stay off the welfare rolls. Leaving their children does not constitute "neglect." Apparently, poor children withstand the rigors of being without their biological mother for eight to ten hours per day better than middle-class children do. "Fathers, on the other hand, have public license (in fact, a veritable public duty) to devote primary attention to job or career" [11]. Sandra and Daryl Bam have illustrated the existent double standard of parental responsibility with the example of a middle-class father who loses his wife: "No matter how much he loved his children, no one would expect him to sacrifice his career in order to stay home with them on a full-time basis — even if he had an independent source of income. No one would charge him with selfishness or lack of parental feeling if he sought professional care for his children during the day" [12].

The facts that nurses mentioned marital and child-rearing responsibilities as precluding employment, that 80 percent of

258 ever-married women under age 45 felt it was better for everyone involved if the man is the achiever outside the home and that women do not believe they should be considered for the best-paying and most responsible jobs suggest that indeed a double standard still exists regarding women and paid employment. These facts also suggest that women, and nurses in particular, lack commitment to roles other than the traditional ones women have always assumed.

"In role selection, a person chooses roles that allow him to behave in a manner compatible with self. A role is chosen because it is associated with expectations for behavior that are congruent with the individual's self-concept and because in that role he would be endowed with attributes like those of his self-concept" [13]. It is still unfortunately true that others' expectations concerning our role behavior are more apt to be based on our sex role than on any other we may choose. This is not so obvious for men as it is for women, because others frequently view men's behavior in terms of their occupation rather than their sex. We rarely hear men described as a male doctor or a male bricklayer. We still frequently hear women described as a woman lawyer, woman doctor or woman truck driver. Until such titles have been eliminated from our language and consciousness, women will, to some extent, be limited in their choices of roles. We *have* reached the point where the opportunities to try new jobs are more available, but society still defines a woman's choice by definition of her sex role.

In order to become a role-breaker, one must have a relatively clear perception of the role that is to be broken. Nurses' role perception and role expectation have been studied by a variety of persons for a variety of reasons. One such study, done in 1960, seems still to have merit in today's social context. Mauksch asserts that: "The theme of internal control which is imposed by the institutional setting of the nurse's work and by the nature of her tasks seems to meet the needs of the person who is in nursing. The nurse serves almost as mother, almost as manager and almost as healer. She navigates between allegiance to the hospital, to the physician and to the patient. She has responsibilities without formal sanctions, and represents many symbols without filling any. This profession in its broad and multiple roles can be called the occupation of 'not quite'" [14]. Are nurses going to continue to allow our profession to be "the occupation of not quite"? There

seems to be a correlation between Mauksch's statement and the
ideas presented by de Beauvoir. Conflict resolution tends to keep
us in the position of being happy or reconciled with a moderate
amount of success. We are satisfied with being not quite managers,
mothers and healers — that is as close as we can allow ourselves
to become successful. If one believes that a role is chosen because
it is associated with expectations for behavior that are congruent
with the individual's self-concept, one must say that the nurse's
self-concept includes factors that allow her to be satisfied with
the "not quite" aspects of nursing. Apparently this is true not
only because empirical evidence shows it to be, but also because
rational thought leads us to the same conclusion. Nurses, mainly
because they are women, have internalized concepts of self that
include satisfaction at being an "almost" person. "Individuals
tend to find continuity in their lives either by means of basic
emphasis on what others have taught them they should do and —
more especially — should not do, or by means of emphasis on
discovering their own lines of direction" [2]. It is now past time
for women, especially those women who are or intend to be
nurses, to discover their own lines of direction.

The question of how one forms one's own lines of direction,
idiom or self-concept — call it what you will — has been recurrent
throughout the ages. There are almost as many theories of how
the process of identification takes place as there are people who
think about it. What makes it possible for some people to be
strong; to endure hostility, frustration and anger; to perceive of
themselves as different and more diversified? What gives some
people the ability or strength to prevail — to hold out and not
give in to society's pressure to conform — to become a deviant?
If our history books can be believed (one does wonder at recorded
history's validity from the perspective of womanhood), Columbus
exhibited somewhat deviant behavior by holding firm to his conviction that the world is round; the Wright brothers were looked
at askance when they insisted man could fly; Margaret Sanger had
to endure more hostility and anger than most people could have
stood because she held firm in her conviction that women have
the right to birth-control information. The list could go on ad
infinitum. The point to be made is that they were role-breakers,
risk-takers — they were different; they marched to a different drummer.

Becoming a Risk-Taker and Role-Breaker

Again, the question is why? Attempts to answer this are complex and varied, but one such attempt concerns the profound subject of *what am I?* According to Lynd, the question of deviance and anomie has been the work of recent social theory, especially the work of Durkheim, Parsons and Merton. "But it remains true that in psychology and in social science in general more attention is still given to adaptation and adjustment to approved social roles and values than to deviation from them. And deviance is far too readily codified in oversimplified terms of genius or of rebellion or, even, of individual pathology" [2]. But can all so-called deviant behavior actually be categorized into genius, rebellion or individual pathology? Was Margaret Sanger just a rebel; was Newton a genius or crazy; was Mary Wollstonecraft just a weird woman who did not fit into her society?

There seem to be indications, according to Lynd, that in some cases a person's sense of self has aspirations that go beyond the demands of society. Some people apparently set requirements for their own behavior that exceed what society demands of them. There have always been prophets, rebels, artists and innovators whose sense of self is related to ideals that they conceive as widely human and at the same time peculiarly their own. The process of attaining a sense of self is a dynamic one that begins with birth and continues, for the most part, until death. Some of us apparently attain a sense of self that we are satisfied with and, as we grow older, become less and less individualistic and more and more a copy formed by pressure from the society in which we live. Adulthood for such people means an ever-increasing need for the protection of being like others. They are less and less inclined to take the risks involved in searching for their own way — in being different. Others of us develop an ever-growing sureness of self in relation to how we "fit" into our world. We become more forthright, more genuinely individual, more willing to take the risk of being different. We are more apt to be interested in discovering the reality of the external world and how that relates or does not relate to the reality of our internal world of self. "The discovery of what is reality in nonpersonal things not related to one's personality is an indispensable part of discovering what is one's personality" [2]. As we go about discovering and creating our self, we involve both our self-image (what one is) and our self-ideal (what one would like to be). The two must be more or less congruent, as well as being congruent with our life-style, in order for us to establish our identity. As long as we can maintain our identity within the confines of the demands of our society, all is well. It is when there is incongruence between what society demands and what our self demands of us that deviant behavior — i.e., role-breaking — is most likely to occur.

Perhaps the most famous example of role-breaking ever recorded is seen in the behavior of Jesus Christ. Whether or not one believes in Christian theology is of no importance here, and there have no doubt been many discussions and dissertations concerning whether Jesus was divinely inspired or merely a man with a strong sense of identity. The point is that He was viewed by most of the people in his society as a role-breaker — a deviant. Today we would be apt to call Him weird, mentally unbalanced or at least somewhat of an eccentric. Most will agree, however, that His aspirations of self went beyond the demands of society. Somewhat closer to contemporary rigors of self-aspiration is Mary Wollstonecraft, whose life is a perfect example of role-breaking. Her book *A Vindication of the Rights of Woman,* written in 1792, argued strongly "that there should be identical education for both boys and girls. It also took the view that the weakness of contemporary women was attributable to their faulty education and social position and urged that special emphasis be given to physical education" [15]. Much of her life and life-style would be viewed even today as somewhat incongruous by most of our society. Even so, she would certainly fit into our life-style better than she did her own. She was independent at age 19, traveled alone extensively, educated herself in several languages, wrote articles and pamphlets that were published without use of a "pen name," had a child out of wedlock, married but did not live in the same house as her husband and is still viewed by some as a deviant. In 1947 she was "analyzed" as being "afflicted with a severe case of penis-envy, an extreme neurotic of the compulsive type" [15]. Rossi goes on to state that it is the fate of pioneers to suffer attacks on their ideas and their personal lives. "What tools are used in these attacks will vary by time and culture: ridicule, social exclusion, damnation, accusation of penis envy, imprisonment, have all been used against those fearless enough to move outside the confines of thought and action approved by

Becoming a Risk-Taker and Role-Breaker

their society. Significant social change does not take place over-night, but through a long series of pressures against the normative boundaries of society" [15].

Another example of a role-breaker and risk-taker who is even closer to us in both time and interest is Margaret Sanger. "From the first issue of her magazine, *Woman Rebel,* in March 1914 to the financial and organizational support she gave to research in hormonal anovulants in the post—World War II period, her life was dedicated to a passionate single-minded commitment to bring the best birth-control methods to ever larger numbers of women around the World" [15]. Her own writings, which are as dramatic as any novel, tell more about her life and herself than anyone's biography of her. The point is, they demonstrate her willingness to pressure society rather than to allow society to pressure her to conform. To be ridiculed, arrested, avoided by other nurses and other women cannot have been a pleasant experience for her, but millions of us have her to thank for our fuller, more rewarding lives. She also left a legacy for every feminist that is epitomized in the following quote taken from her book *Woman and the New Race:* "The woman is not needed to do man's work. She is not needed to think man's thoughts. She need not fear that the masculine mind, almost universally dominant, will fail to take care of its own. Her mission is not to enhance the masculine spirit, but to express the feminine; hers is not to preserve a man-made world, but to create a human world by the infusion of the feminine element into all of its activities" [15].

To bring the examples of role-breakers even closer, today's woman and nurse only has to look around to find nurses who are willingly bearing the cost of being considered deviant. One such role-breaker is Rena Murtha, Director of Nursing Services for New York City Prison Health Services. In the October 1974 issue of *The American Nurse,* the official newspaper of the American Nurses' Association, Ms. Murtha is quoted as being proud of the innovations she has established in order to provide health care for the inmates of the eleven prisons in New York City. Not the least of these innovations is a nurse ombudsman who serves the prison system. "She is probably the only nurse advocate for prisoners in the country," said Ms. Murtha [16]. I would say that both Ms. Murtha and the unnamed nurse ombudsman are role-breakers. Another example, also taken from *The American Nurse* [17], is Ruth Murphy, the American Nurses' Association's first honorary Nurse Practitioner. Ms. Murphy provides health care for the people of Elk County, Kansas, and has for the past seven years. Collaboration with physicians is no longer a problem for her. While she is referring patients to physicians, they are referring patients to her for long-term, continuing care.

In giving examples of nurses who are now role-breakers and risk-takers, I would be remiss if I did not mention the nurses who are in training for the space program, which had been limited to men up to the time of their entry into it. There were feelings that the rigorous training needed to be an astronaut as well as the unknown hazards of space travel were too dangerous for women. Women and nurses should be doubly proud that not only has our space program managed to change that attitude, but it has admitted nurses into training to become the first women space travelers.

This list of role-breakers would not be in any way complete if I did not mention thousands of nurses who are unknown or nameless to me: nurse-midwives, family nurse practitioners, pediatric nurse practitioners, family-planning nurse practitioners, adult nurse practitioners — in other words, all of us who are filling the gaps in the health care system, all of us who are strong enough to demand that patient care be more than "a pill to cure all ills," all of us who see ourselves as patient care advocates before we see ourselves as nurses or by any other title.

This chapter has been an effort to portray some of the joys and frustrations of being a role-breaker. If I have spent more time on the negative aspects of taking risks and breaking roles, it is not because I do not enjoy doing both, but it is important for those who are considering becoming role-breakers to be aware that the costs are high. The rewards, of course, are worth it. How can one describe the exhilarating, awesome fear one experiences when the realization comes that, as the primary health care provider, one is accountable and responsible for the health of some six thousand patients! I would be less than honest if I did not say there is a certain sense of joy and power in being able to refer a patient to a physician whom she and I have chosen together as the one most likely to meet her needs. When women seek me out to help them solve a health problem, pick the best kind of contraception or advise them on medical care, this boosts my ego. I feel a great sense of fulfillment when I have managed to do any of these well or when a patient tells me that her experience in my clinic is the first time she has ever sought out health care without feeling degraded, embarrassed, ignorant or a nuisance. I also feel that the "nurse-doctor game" is surely dying when I can consult with a physician on the level of two professionals trying to solve a patient's problem and the physician says, "Thanks for calling me" or "Thanks for referring the patient." Those kinds of remarks lead me to believe that physicians are slowly but surely becoming more amenable toward an expanding role for nurses. It is within memory that no physician would dream of accepting a referral from anyone other than another physician.

Both professions are changing in their role-concepts and role-behaviors. In the not too distant future those of us who are now perceived as role-breakers will be seen as maintainers of the status quo, and the risk-takers of that age will be urging us to break the chains that bind us to the past. Until that age is here, the nursing profession must increase still more the growing numbers of nurses who are the present-day risk-takers, so that we can overwhelm (with sheer numbers if nothing else) those among our own profession and other health professions who cling to the unreal roles of the past. "Professions are subject to the same deadening forces that affect all other human institutions: an attachment to time-honored ways, reverence for established procedures, a preoccupation with one's own vested interests, and an excessively narrow definition of what is relevant and important" [18]. Health care for this country may well rest on our ability as role-breakers to change those "deadening forces."

References

1. Janeway, Elizabeth. *Man's World, Woman's Place: A Study in Social Mythology.* New York: Dell, 1971.
2. Lynd, Helen Merrell. Shame, Guilt, and Identity Beyond Roles. In *The Self in Social Interaction,* Vol. I, Gordon, Chad, and Gergen, Kenneth J. (Eds.). New York: Wiley, 1968.
3. de Beauvoir, Simone. *The Second Sex.* New York: Vintage — Random House, 1952. (Translated and edited by H. M. Parshley, 1974.)

4. Stanton, Marjorie. Political Action and Nursing. *Nursing Clinics of North America,* Vol. 9, No. 3, September 1974.
5. Lambertson, Eleanor. The Changing Role of Nursing and Its Regulation. *Nursing Clinics of North America,* Vol. 9, No. 3, September 1974, pp. 395–402.
6. Hinsvark, Inez. Implications for Acting in the Expanded Role of the Nurse. *Nursing Clinics of North America,* Vol. 9, No. 3, September 1974, pp. 411–423.
7. Chesler, Phyllis. *Women and Madness.* New York: Avon, 1972.
8. Keller, Nancy. The Nurse's Role: Is It Expanding or Shrinking? In *The Expanded Role of the Nurse,* Browning, Mary, and Lewis, Edith P. (Eds.). New York: The American Journal of Nursing Company, 1973.
9. Norris, Catherine M. Direct Access to the Patient. In *Changing Patterns of Nursing Practice,* Lewis, Edith P. (Ed.). New York: The American Journal of Nursing Company, 1971.
10. McCormick, Regina, and Crawford, Ronald. Attitudes of Professional Nurses Toward Primary Care. *Nursing Research,* Vol. 18, No. 6, November–December, 1969.
11. Women Accept Some Sex Stereotypes but Favor Greater Equality with Men. *Family Planning Digest,* Vol. 3, No. 1, January 1974. The Bureau of Community Health Services, Health Services Administration, Department of Health, Education and Welfare.
12. Bam, Sandra, and Bam, Daryl, as quoted by Polatnick, Margaret. Why Men Don't Rear Children: A Power Analysis. *Berkeley Journal of Sociology,* Vol. 18, 1973.
13. Blackman, Carl W., and Secord, Paul F. The Self and Role Selection. In *The Self in Social Interaction,* Vol. I, Gordon, Chad, and Gergen, Kenneth J. (Eds.). New York: Wiley, 1968.
14. Mauksch, Hans O. *The Nurse: A Study in Role Perception.* Abstract of an unpublished dissertation submitted to the Department of Sociology, The University of Chicago, April 1960.
15. Rossi, Alice S. (Ed.). *The Feminist Papers from Adams to de Beauvoir.* New York: Bantam, 1973.
16. *The American Nurse.* Vol. 6, No. 10, October 1974. The American Nurses' Association, Kansas City, Mo.
17. *The American Nurse.* Vol. 6, No. 7, July 1974. The American Nurses' Association, Kansas City, Mo.
18. Gardner, J. W. *No Easy Victories,* Rowan, Helen (Ed.). New York: Harper & Row, 1968, p. 42.

10 Success and Antisuccess—

Marlene Grissum

There is nothing as exciting or as wonderful as choosing a difficult goal, working hard and succeeding [1].
David Viscott

The Dichotomy of Woman

Success can be defined as the ability to function in a chosen profession with some measure of peer recognition [2]. Commonly, there is also a sense of accomplishment; a feeling of having attained a goal, of having attained one's desired end. It is not unusual to hear successful men described in terms of their occupational role, while women are defined as successful in terms of their sex role. If women are defined as successful in terms of occupation, most often it goes something like this: "She's a good lawyer — for a woman," or "She's an excellent manager — and she's pretty, too." In other words, successful women are viewed, particularly by men, as somewhat of an oddity, as if some freak accident of nature had created an extra species that was neither masculine (rightfully successful) nor feminine (rightfully antisuccessful).

When I speak of antisuccessful I do not mean *un*successful. People who are antisuccessful have not tried and failed — they have not, or cannot, try at all. The concept is similar to what Matina Horner, a sociologist and president of Radcliffe College, calls *success avoidance*. The difference between successful people and antisuccessful people most likely lies in their motivational differences. Successful women, and men, probably have sufficiently gratified their basic needs for safety, love, respect and self-esteem so that they are motivated by trends that lead them toward growth. Antisuccessful people are so involved with gratifying their basic needs for love, respect, safety and self-esteem that they cannot be outwardly motivated. Their needs for belonging, for love relations, for respect can only be satisfied by others. In other words, they are dependent people. They dare not be growth-motivated because in their dependent position they are not really in control of their own fate. They must be beholden to the sources of supply of needed gratification and be sensitive to other people's approval, affection and good will. Maslow says of such people: "Their wishes, their whims, their rules and laws govern him [her] and must be appeased lest he [she] jeopardize his [her] sources of supply" [3]. Because the motivation of antisuccessful people is dependent upon others, they are afraid to try for fear of failing. If they fail, they have proved themselves unworthy of the love and respect they must have for gratification. They are also afraid to try because they might succeed. Success might put them in jeopardy of displeasing the persons they depend on. In other words, their feeling is that no one loves a loser *or* a winner.

In contrast, persons who are growth-motivated try to increase their own potential. They view growth as fulfillment — the degree or measure of attaining one's desired end — success. They reach gratification through self-development. They are less likely to be dependent on others to meet their needs and more likely to feel capable of, and find more pleasure in, meeting their own needs. Their need gratification is *not* dependent on others. They respect themselves; have self-esteem; are motivated primarily by trends to self-actualization [3]. Instead of being afraid to try, they are eager for opportunities. Growth motivation is desired and welcomed, enjoyable and pleasant. Gratification leads to a desire for more growth, which leads to an increased feeling of excitement for more stimulation. In fact, it could be said of success-oriented people that "Growth is, in itself, a rewarding and exciting process" [3].

What about women? Are they growth-motivated or motivated by basic needs? What makes women growth-motivated? What makes women oriented by basic need? Are there any successful

By attempting to answer the first question, the next three will
be answered as well. *So,* what about women? Are they success-
or antisuccess-oriented? One would have to answer that, for the
most part, women are antisuccess-oriented. For instance, the
human characteristics that are most likely to be used to describe
women are passive, dependent, tender, loving, self-sacrificing.
To illustrate the point: in a survey [4] to determine the "average
housewife," a Haug Associates (Los Angeles) survey team determined that the average housewife, among other characteristics,
"has little interest or skill to explore or probe." She is open to
suggestions and guidance that fit her needs. She doesn't use too
much energy on long-term goals but is day-to-day oriented. She
"finds satisfaction in a small world, the center of which is her
home." She "experiences confusion and discomfort when faced
with ambiguity or too many alternatives." And, she "feels that
mental activity is arduous." Now, one must keep in mind that this
survey was done by men for men in order to further their careers
in advertising. Not for one moment do I believe there are really
women who would fit this "average housewife" stereotype. Most
housewives I know have every right to be highly indignant with
such a composite picture. There are, no doubt, women who do
fit *some* parts of this, but I believe there are also men who fit *some*
of it as well. For instance, there are men and women who like to
watch TV rather than read (another characteristic given for housewives), and who *doesn't* experience a sense of confusion and discomfort when faced with ambiguity or too many alternatives?
Because people perceive that women have some or all of these
characteristics, they also perceive that women are dependent —
requiring basic need gratification through others, and therefore
cannot succeed or, even worse, do not want to try to succeed.
The composite picture of women as shown in this particular survey
is that of a child or perhaps a well-behaved house dog. Nevertheless, if it is true that motivation is either self-controlled or other-
controlled, and if it is true that dependent people are motivated
by others, we must look at the composite of the "average housewife" as having some truth buried within its sexist heart. The
socialization process that women go through tends to make them

passive, dependent people with low levels of self-esteem. Most women are raised to believe that their primary fulfillment will be attained through others. They validate themselves through their husbands and children. To some extent they live vicariously.

Contrast this with how Allport describes people who are "active experiencing" [3]. Active experiencing results in physical, emotional and intellectual self-involvement. There is recognition and further exploration of one's abilities. The person initiates creative activity. At the same time, the person is finding out about her own pace or rhythm, how much of a task she can assume, and she learns to avoid taking on too much. Through active experiencing, the person gains in skills that can be applied to other experiences and she has an opportunity to find out what she is interested in. It is true that some women find satisfaction in the small world of their home. There is no reason to believe, however, that active experiencing cannot occur in a small world, and finding satisfaction there is not limited to passive, dependent women. Apparently, most people find satisfaction in the small world of their home; otherwise, there would not be so many of them! When the *need* for that satisfaction is dependent upon others for fulfillment, however, we are focusing upon basic-need motivation. The need for safety, love and respect can be satisfied only by other people — and because of our socialization, women have not grown past the stage of having basic needs fulfilled. The whole idea of growth is an extremely complex one and is not the basis for this book; however, women need to know at least the rudiments of how growth occurs in order to understand our own arrested development in some areas. In terms of a child's growth and development, "growth takes place when the next step forward is subjectively more delightful, more joyful, more intrinsically satisfying than the previous gratification with which we have become familiar" [3]. The child tends to try out his or her powers, to test and manipulate the world. When satiated with that level of testing or manipulating, the child will attempt the next level. Maslow uses the example of a toddler testing out a new room or place. First the child explores the room with her eyes, next with a few steps away from her protection — her parent. Slowly but surely the distance grows ever wider between herself and her security. Now, if the parent — the security — leaves the room, the child immediately becomes anxious and probably will regress to crawling instead of walking. In other words, within all people there are forces which urge us to be motivated toward self-actualization as well as forces which urge us backward toward a lower level of safety and security. So one set of forces keeps us afraid to take chances, afraid of independence, freedom and separateness, while the other set forces us forward toward confidence, full functioning of all capacities and self-actualization or attainment.

There seems to be a correlation between what Maslow has to say about the growth of children and the idea of women and success. Maslow asserts that if a child "is forced to stay at the simple level he gets bored and restless with what formerly delighted him. He *wants* to go on, to move, to grow. Only if frustration, failure, disapproval, ridicule come at the next step does he fixate or regress" [3]. I believe that women have wanted to go on, to grow past the dependent, passive persons that many of them are. Some have indeed done just that; however, others have been arrested in their development and have become antisuccessful. The set of forces that pushes them backward to safety and security is stronger than the forces that push them forward toward self-fulfillment. The antisuccessful women are those who continue to meet with frustration, failure, disapproval and ridicule and so have become fixated or have regressed in their development of self. An element of courage is needed in order to create success, whether that "success" is your first step or your first job. "Thus to discover in oneself a great talent can certainly bring exhilaration, but it also brings a fear of the dangers and responsibilities and duties of being a leader and of being all alone" [3].

These fears are among the forces that keep women antisuccessful. Many women have been socialized to believe that to probe, to search, to discover, to create, to affirm are masculine activities; to do any of them will defeminize them. So many women never grow past the stage of needing their basic needs met. They must have their own self-esteem affirmed rather than affirming it themselves through further knowledge and growth. They must have their need for love reaffirmed verbally and behaviorally by those whom they serve rather than learning the significance of self-love. They must have their sense of worth affirmed through others by serving others rather than learning self-worth through growth. The whole idea of self-affirmation through others is incongruent with the idea of success. To accomplish, attain, prosper, to reach one's desired end depends on self-motivation — there must be an inner force or desire that pushes the person toward growth. Self-affirmation through others is therefore extremely congruent with the whole idea of antisuccess. The woman who has become fixated or has regressed to the point where her primary motivational force is to have her dependency needs met by others dares not use any energy in aiming for a goal that is *higher* than her basic needs for love, respect and safety. She has no courage to begin. Fear of failure is ingrained in many people. They lack energy and courage to try to learn from failure, to overcome it by creating something new [5].

If the idea of success-antisuccess can be accepted as a theory with some validity, we must still look at the question: What makes a woman motivated by basic needs and what makes a woman growth-motivated? There is no simple answer to either question. The answers are so complex, in fact, that they may not be answers; they may be only surmises. We can merely make conjectures based on the scanty evidence of personal observation and a search for possible answers. "Because women are socialized to be dependent" seems to be the first part of the answer to the question of what makes us motivated by basic needs. As we grow up, it is impressed on us that we are not capable of growth beyond the basic-needs level. It is as if society is saying that women are not worthy of higher levels of growth — that we do not need to be motivated toward success because we will not be doing anything that can be judged as successful. Growth motivation is, in many ways, dependent upon intelligence, and women are socialized to believe that they are not as intelligent as men. In fact, we grow up believing that not only are we incapable of any sustained intellectual effort, but that we should not even try because it is displeasing to those who will supply us with basic need gratification.

There are women now who have broken out of the confines dictated by society, but they are often feared and rejected by men and derogated by nonliberated women who are threatened or envious of what they have done. In one survey, two researchers presented biographical sketches of four extremely competent women to 48 men and 48 women students. The sketches represented

depicted as either competitive or noncompetitive) and masculine
or feminine sex role preference. "Although women of both sex-
role preferences were portrayed as equally success-oriented, the
students felt the woman with the masculine bent was more ambitious, indicating that 'success orientation is, to some extent,
perceived as an intrinsic part of the masculine sex role' say the
researchers" [6]. In essence, the 96 students could be said to be
representative of our society in that they reconfirmed the stereotypic image that portrays women as masculine if they are ambitious
or successful. Horner points out in her study regarding success
and women that women are basically afraid of success. In fact,
she found that our society views success in a woman as deviant
behavior. In most societies, including our own, deviants are
ostracized, banished, feared and/or ridiculed. Is it any wonder that
women experience a fear of success, that they are antisuccess-
oriented, particularly when we consider that all of us have a need
to be loved and respected by others in order to love and respect
ourselves?

Success-oriented people have apparently had their need for love
met enough times at enough levels so that they no longer have to
be totally dependent on others. They have experienced love from
others enough so that they have learned how to love and respect
themselves. Thus, they can afford to take the risk of being successful and being ostracized, banished, feared or ridiculed; they do
not have to be totally dependent on others to validate themselves.
The reverse, of course, is true of women who are antisuccessful.
They have never had their needs for love and respect fulfilled
enough to learn to love and respect themselves and still are totally
dependent on others to fulfill them. Consequently, they dare not
risk being ostracized, banished and ridiculed because they have
very little self-esteem to depend on. Involved in the problem is the
idea that women are socialized to believe that they should not be
dominant, as dominance is generally viewed as a male characteristic.
In order to be successful, it is oftentimes necessary to use dominance
in the sense of taking command or leading others. Women are
programmed to take commands rather than give them, part of the
feminine characteristic of passivity. The most obvious aspect of
what makes women growth-motivated is that it is the same forces

that make men growth-motivated. The rare women who are growth-motivated have been allowed to develop along independent, free lines. In comparing the similar characteristics of successful women in the sciences, Kundsin [2] found that they all established their successful careers without societal support, all needed and received parental support and all were influenced to believe that education and the attainment of knowledge are as important for women as for men. The most significant finding that was established at this particular conference on successful women was that there is a real need for parental support, from both parents. All the participants felt this was imperative in order to develop the self-esteem and self-confidence needed to succeed. This seems to add credence to Maslow's stance that growth motivation is an inherent part of the self-actualization process.

In most instances, women are socialized not to be self-actualizing people. They are urged to consider whether or not they are doing the right thing and whether or not their actions will be pleasing to others. Being involved in pleasing others and doing the right thing usually means they will not allow themselves to be motivated toward growth and will not use their energies to develop their own potentials. Successful women, however, do use their energies for self-development. Apparently, they have been encouraged and fulfilled by the significant others in their lives to the extent that they no longer need to be passive and dependent or fearful that they will destroy their source of need-fulfillment. They have become sufficiently autonomous to depend on their inner strengths to carry them through the stresses of making important life decisions, experiencing the anxiety of competition and the fear of being ostracized by society. Of course, men also face many of the same problems, but men have society's approval to succeed while women do not, especially in occupational roles. Success for women is more acceptable today than it has ever been, but even women who are described as *highly* successful are usually found at the bottom of the top. A survey done by *Fortune* magazine in 1972 indicated that men outnumbered women 600 to 1 in very high positions in large American corporations. If a measure of success is the money one is paid (and our society uses that as the primary measurement), again, women are not often found in highly successful positions. In the same survey *Fortune* found that out of some

Women have traditionally been kept off the ladder of success
for reasons that clearly are invalid. In many instances the reasons
have been discriminatory, clearly male-oriented, in that women
who compete threaten men. There are now laws against sex-based
discrimination, and women have an opportunity to press forward
toward success in any field they choose. Unless they have been
socialized to be growth-motivated, though, it still seems unlikely
that they will assume the mantle of success with any regularity.
Little girls need motivation from significant others; this motivation
will push them toward growth. They need to learn that they can
compete with men and still maintain a sense of self-worth that is
free from guilt. At the same time, men will have to learn, from
childhood, how to compete with women and how to lose to women
without also losing their sense of self-worth. They will have to
learn that it does not detract from their masculinity to compete
with women, just as women will have to learn that it does not
decrease their femininity to compete with men. Men will have to
find some other means of boosting their ego than the still-acceptable
idea that they are superior to women. Women will have to find
some different means of defining themselves rather than through
others; particularly, they will have to destroy the concept that
they are inferior and therefore not as worthy of attaining success
simply because they happen to be women.

Men are motivated to achieve primarily because from childhood
on they are *taught* to achieve, to be proud of their growth, to be
goal-oriented, to be outward-reaching individuals. They are not
expected to conform, to be passive, to let others define what is
acceptable behavior or set boundaries for them to nearly the
extent that women are. When one investigates what makes women
growth-motivated, it is almost always that they too have been
encouraged and taught that achievement is their right and responsibility. It is not unusual to hear a successful person describe his
own ability to succeed in terms of having always believed that
success was possible. Needless to say, parents have a large part to
do with this attitude or belief. Probably the most frequent remark
of successful people is "My parents always told me I could be
anything I wanted to be." It is a discouraging thought that so

much potential talent for success in women has been shut off, diverted or channeled into frustration because parents did not include their daughters when they said "You can be *anything*." In light of the fact that women have been tuned-out, turned-off and generally ignored by the vast majority of parents regarding their need for success or their potential for it, it is amazing that there are as many successful women as there are. Of course the numbers depend on how one defines success, but even with a structured, limited definition of success that includes those aspects listed at the beginning of this chapter, one would still have to answer yes to the question: "Are there any successful women?" If we speak in terms of the ability to function in a chosen profession with some measure of peer recognition, we can then include a far larger number of women. Nevertheless, even if we speak in terms of accomplishments — of attaining a desired end — in a recognized field or occupation, there are still some women who could be classified as successful.

In our society, however, occupational excellence (or success) is not enough for women to be considered truly successful — we must demonstrate competency in a wide range of roles. For instance, one characteristic shared by all 12 women cited in *Women and Success* was that they were or had been married and raised families. We must be competent mothers and wives as well as competent in our occupational choice before society will consider us successful. Of course, this is not so for men — they can be totally incompetent as fathers and husbands and still be considered extremely successful persons. Until society accepts the idea that child-rearing is the responsibility of both parents, women will continue to have their occupational success, or the lack of it, judged on other criteria than just their ability to perform their job. Until men assume their equal responsibilities in child-rearing and give up the myth that because only women can have babies only women can rear them, women will have fewer opportunities to achieve success in their chosen occupation. A man's primary goal is almost always oriented toward success in his job. Nearly all his energy is directed toward that end. It is sad that our society has seen fit to socialize men to occupational goal achievement to the exclusion of all other goals and relationships. By doing so, we have perpetuated the process from one generation

to the next and we have missed opportunities for developing
women's talents for success and men's talents for nurturing,
compassion and tenderness — which can also be considered
characteristics of success.

The same social control system that prepares a man to achieve
in the occupation of his choice undermines a woman's abilities
to do so because it does not sanction commitment and ambition
for women unless that dedication and ambition are for others. It
is acceptable for a woman to have a strong sense of commitment
to further her husband's career, but in many instances it is unacceptable for her to have the same urge to further her own. It
is perfectly all right for a woman to be ambitious for her children,
particularly her male children. But society does not sanction
ambition in women when it is to achieve their own ends and will
"punish" them for it by viewing them as masculine and not good
mothers or wives. Only the most elite of women, the "queen
bees" for instance, are allowed by society to be committed to
and ambitious for their own success.

Very rarely, if ever, are women encouraged in their efforts for
success through the informal but extremely effective method that
Epstein calls "the creation of competence" [8]. In many occupational fields, competence is developed by exposing a new person to
"inside" information. He is taught how to avoid pitfalls and is
given access to powerful people and information to help develop
his potentials. Thus competence is created by this route of on-the-
job training that is given only to select individuals who important
gatekeepers — the people in the profession with power — decide
are capable, those who have the necessary talent and perseverance
to continue their striving for success. Because almost all the
important gatekeepers are men, they are more likely to choose
men as the persons with the greatest chance to become competent;
women are less likely to be chosen because they do not fit the
image of competence in our society. Even if they are allowed into
the inner circle, they will probably be considered less successful
than the men in the inner circle. Epstein contends that this is
secondary to the fact that women are not subjected to the disciplines of their profession in the same manner that men are. They
are often rewarded for *any* level of performance because for a
woman to do even just an adequate job appears unique. Also,

women are usually perceived as a class, and their deficiencies are viewed as belonging to *all* women rather than to individuals. They are considered successful with less effort because they are "graded" by a different standard than men are. Because women are generally perceived as being less competent, they are more likely to be rewarded for irrelevant behaviors or to be ignored. This knowledge that they are on the periphery, that they are more likely to stay at the bottom of the top, undermines their motivation to achieve in their profession or occupation. Because of these perceptions, plus the socialization process, women do not compete — they rarely put their talents and capacities to the test. They do not believe that they can succeed or fail on their own merits and contributions. Are there successful women? Yes, there are; but they are a scarce commodity, and in reality, society sets rather severe limitations even on them.

I have taken the stand that there are successful women, and since almost all nurses are women, it would seem that at least some of the successful women of the world should or could be nurses. Are there any successful nurses? That again depends on the definition of success and on who is doing the defining. For instance, if peer recognition is part of our definition of success, we must first define *peer*. Does peer mean those nurses with whom we work on a daily basis? Does peer mean nurses with the same educational background who are doing nursing in the same general area? Does peer mean the whole sisterhood of nurses who make up the profession of nursing? I suppose that my definition of peer can involve any or all of these levels of nurses, depending on the situation in which any one nurse is involved. If we receive some measure of peer recognition from our own work group and they define us as successful nurses, we have at least attained that small amount of success. If we are recognized by our peer group — meaning those with similar education and work goals — as an excellent nurse, we have reached another plateau of success. And, if we are recognized by the larger society of nurses as an outstanding leader in nursing, an excellent nurse, we have attained another level. The level of success that we as nurses attain and aspire to is dependent upon our inner motivation, just as it is with any other person who seeks success.

There is however, another group who judge nurses as successful or unsuccessful, and that is the patients they are taking care of. Just as in any other service occupation or profession, nurses must be accountable to the patients they are responsible for. If we cannot deliver effective, worthwhile care to patients, it isn't really likely that we will be successful, no matter how much peer recognition we receive. Ultimately, our success or lack of it is dependent upon whether patients perceive that we are excellent in our field. However, the messages are pretty clear as to what our patients feel about nursing as a whole, and it is not favorable. In general, they are as disillusioned with the nursing care they receive as they are with the medical care and the high cost of being sick or trying to maintain a state of health. When one hears former patients give testimonials to the fact that they rarely if ever saw a registered nurse while in the hospital, one wonders whether or not there are really any successful nurses. When one observes a maternity ward where the *only* time a registered nurse ever enters a postpartum patient's room is to give her a pill, one wonders if there are any nurses who really want to be successful. When one hears an entire nursing staff of an ambulatory care unit define nursing care in terms of assisting physicians, one wonders whether there are any nurses who really even know what nursing is.

What or who sets up the mechanisms that are responsible for this? Are some of those mechanisms unique to our profession? Or are they the same mechanisms, disguised by nursing's private vocabulary and sense of separateness, that keep all women on the fringes of attaining a complete measure of success?

The bureaucratic system of health care in our contemporary society is certainly partly responsible for the opinions nurses have of their work. To illustrate the point, we need only to consider what happens to an "average" new graduate in her first job. To begin with, she is offered a salary that should be considered an insult to her intelligence, but will not be because she has nothing with which to compare it. In January 1972, the American Nurses' Association's statistics department reported the average starting salary for a new graduate in a staff nurse position was $8,200 per year [9]. She then may be put to work in the area of her choice but more likely will be assigned wherever the hospital needs her. Very little consideration is given to her area of expertise, interest or specialty training. In other words, she becomes a worker, a drone in a bureaucratic system that for the most part ignores her. The hospital hierarchy, including the nursing service department, pays little heed to the fact that they have hired a professional person, one who has spent various numbers of years in preparation. There would be quite a furor if a hospital hired a physician whose specialty was cardiovascular medicine and then put him to work in surgery. Nevertheless, it often happens to nurses, whether they are new graduates or just new to a particular hospital.

The next step in the new graduate's "orientation" to the real world of nursing is her realization that she cannot practice as she was taught! There is just *no way* she can provide individualized care for 30 or 40 patients when she is the only registered nurse working that shift — hence, patients' complaints that they never even see registered nurses in the hospital. In fact, she will be somewhat of a supernurse if she can even manage to learn what kind of care other people are providing "her" patients with. The inability to keep up with what is going on with patients she is responsible for is a direct result of the fact that she is expected to perform non-nursing functions by the score, plus the fact that the number of nurses and non-nurses on any one unit is so small as to be ridiculous as well as dangerous, particularly on evening and night shifts. Needless to say, the nurse is expected to rotate shifts! After all, hospitals have to stay open twenty-four hours, seven days a week. There is little or no consideration of any plan for work scheduling except the traditional 7 AM to 3 PM, 3 PM to 11 PM and 11 PM to 7 AM schedule.

Is it any wonder that she begins to view herself as an entity, a cog in the wheel, an ineffectual housekeeper who is responsible for almost everything and to almost everyone except those (the patients) for whom she is supposed to be doing all this? Whether or not her peers recognize her as an excellent nurse — and they may, particularly if she does not make waves — she will see herself as unsuccessful, a failure. Patients will not see her at all, either figuratively or literally, but they are likely to see *all* nurses as unsuccessful. After an indeterminate amount of time, she will make one of two choices: She may opt to leave nursing and will probably be lost to the profession, a good nurse who could not take the hassles involved, a potentially successful woman who got out of a dangerous situation. But she will probably feel like a failure for having done so. Or her choice may be to "hang in there" until those in the nursing hierarchy notice her and decide that she deserves to be rewarded because she is a good nurse. So, she will get promoted to be head nurse, where she has even less contact with patients. Until very recently, joining the hierarchy of nursing management was the only reward route open to nurses. There seems to be a paradox here. A system that rewards a nurse for providing good nursing care by "advancing" her further and further away from the patient who needs and wants her has a very strange view of success! Furthermore, there has been very little financial reward for the nurse's advancement. The average head nurse made less than $10,000 per year in 1972, and even directors of nursing rarely made over $20,000. So by most standards, these nurses cannot be called a success.

What keeps them there if they have little reward financially and even less professionally? Epstein, describing women in general, believes that in part women are persuaded into having a high level of commitment by rewards that are sex-role directed rather than occupational-role directed [8]. They are more likely to be rewarded with affection and attention than with money, rank or power. These rewards (attention and affection) are more apt to generate commitment to a person (a doctor or the director of nursing), a group of persons (the nursing service department) or an institution (the hospital) than to a profession or a discipline. In essence, women (and nurses) are rewarded for irrelevant performance or they are ignored. In any hospital hierarchy where nurses can *only* be rewarded by advancing away from direct access to the patient, they are being rewarded for irrelevant performance. They may very well be described as successful by their peers, but are they? It seems to me that there must be a way to measure success in terms of how those we serve view success.

Perhaps one measure of success for nurses by those we serve can be identified in those settings where nurses are the primary health providers. One such setting is Loeb Center for Nursing and Rehabilitation in the Bronx in New York. Loeb Center, started approximately eleven years ago, was a new concept then and still is to a great degree. This is exemplified by the fact that nurses staff its administration, provide all direct patient care and have the final word on who is admitted and when patients are discharged.

It could be said that the success of Loeb Center is a reflection of the success of Ms. Lydia Hall, who developed, planned and directed the whole idea. That others consider it successful can be seen in the facts that physicians refer more and more patients every year, Blue Cross has decreased its rate of cost to half what they charge other affiliated hospitals and patients actively encourage their physicians to refer them there. Professional nursing is the most important aspect of care the patients receive there. Medicine and other disciplines are secondary to nursing care, and nursing is in charge of the total plan of care for each patient. Part of every patient's plan of care involves discharge planning, which involves the nurse, the physician and the patient. Professional nurses provide all the nursing care given to any patient at Loeb Center. Genrose Alfono, the present director, believes that this center is only one way to reverse the trend of "advancing" nurses away from patients. For twenty-odd years, Ms. Alfono said, "nurses have not been accountable for their own practice, because there were just too many people involved — LPNs, aides, orderlies, physicians. We've demonstrated just one way of reversing that trend" [10].

Another example of a setting where nurses are primary health care providers and can therefore measure their success by how their patients see them is the ambulatory health care agency. In many different kinds of ambulatory settings, nurses are now doing physical, psychological and social assessments on healthy or stabilized chronically ill patients and providing the patients with whatever assistance they need in maintaining their state of health. Family planning agencies are typical settings in which nurses are now responsible for providing the major part of care for healthy adult women who need education and assistance in family planning and maintaining health. One measure of success for these nurses may be by patients referring other women in need of care to that agency. Word of mouth is probably still one of the fastest, most efficient methods of communication. When patients perceive the care they receive as a positive experience, they are likely to tell others about that experience. One of the questions asked by our agency on a self-administered entry questionnaire is: "Where did you hear about our agency?" Research I have done indicates that greater than 60 percent of our new patients are referred there by present or former patients. Certainly other variables are involved, including cost, the amount of waiting time before an appointment and the amount of time spent in the clinic, to name a few. If nurses can keep down the cost to the patient and minimize waiting time for appointments and time spent in the clinic, these too can be used as a measure of our success, since they are three variables that patients complain a great deal about. When we take these variables into account, plus the fact that the patient will not be seeing a physician (which can be viewed as positive or negative by the patient) and we still have a percentage greater than half, it seems that this could be used as a measure of success for nurses providing the care.

This should not necessarily be construed as a reflection on medical care, even though women are beginning to make loud, unhappy noises about much of the care they receive from physicians. It is not unusual for women to tell me about their experiences with male physicians, particularly in instances when they were seeking health care and had no illness. They frequently tell me they have never had an examination in which the physician told them *what* was being done, *why* it was being done or the results. They seldom receive adequate education concerning self-care such as a self-administered breast examination. Many do not receive either — a breast examination or education on how to do one themselves. It is not unusual for patients to be sent home from a visit with a doctor with no instruction on how to use the contraceptive he prescribed, what to expect as side-effects or what *kind* it is. In other words, patients tell me they receive no education, have little or no chance to ask questions and leave feeling they have no right to complain to the person who did not meet their needs. However, nurses' success should not then imply that physicians are therefore unsuccessful. It is analogous to comparing apples and oranges. They are entirely different but equally important. And nurses and doctors should be aware of that difference as much as patients are. This awareness can also be a measure of our success — if we can actually become a team in meeting patients' health or illness needs, all three members of the team (patient, nurse and doctor) can be viewed as successful.

In more and more instances, the team concept is beginning to be actualized. As Lambertson points out, the idea of team does

284 not have to be structured in time and place [11]. Collaboration between the physician and the nurse saves the patient and the health care personnel time and money, and it provides a better kind of health-illness care. In many instances, it is better utilization of education and skills by far for the nurse to be responsible and accountable for the *health* care a patient needs, while being a liaison for the patient in situations in which illness is involved. Most physicians provide excellent illness care but have little time or interest in being primarily responsible for health care. They are quite willing to share the responsibility of health care with qualified nurses because it gives them more time to devote to illness care, while at the same time assuring well patients that they are not being neglected. When put into this perspective, most doctors and nurses can see that the team concept is not a threat to either's self-esteem, and more importantly it provides an opportunity for patients to receive better care. Certainly, there are other characteristics of a team as well as other health care providers who are part of the team; but the fact remains that patients are more likely to seek help from either nurses or physicians first. The best help we can provide is referral to someone who can meet the patient's need better than we can. In my own practice I refer patients to a variety of health care providers, including nutritionists, social workers, community workers, teachers, other nurses and lawyers. In other words, I call upon a broad range of personnel, constituting all possible resources, and those personnel could be called a health care team. The abilities to recognize the patient's needs, know the community in which you work, know the mechanics involved in referring a patient to another person or agency and knowing how to educate the patient in utilizing the other agency constitutes one measure of success for nurses involved in direct, primary care to patients.

Research is another area where nurses are successful. Their success may not be viewed by clients as directly affecting them; the end-results of almost all nursing research, however, can be applied in one way or another to improve the quality of care nurses provide. Nursing research is not new — nurses have been involved in many research projects. Often though, this has been research aimed at solving a medical problem or some aspect of treatment of a disease rather than research involving nursing care.

But for the past decade or so, nurses have been endeavoring 285
through research to find avenues for improving the profession,
and the results of nursing research are now being disseminated and
put to use, particularly by those nurses who are interested in improving their own practice and the image of nursing. As nursing
education has become less oriented toward apprenticeship and
more directed toward a solid foundation in basic sciences, the
humanities and scientific inquiry, nurses began to recognize the
need for research into definitive methods to improve nursing
practice. Until recently, a lack of research had left nurses dependent
on stereotyped techniques and procedures that were probably
interpreted differently by each individual. Since there were no
valid means of assessing the effects of our interventions, it was
nearly impossible to define what we meant by optimum care.
Research can give us a body of knowledge, or a set of probabil-
ities, to guide nursing care. Nursing research has been extremely
limited, however, and most of it has been directed toward issues
in education and professionalism rather than toward clinical
practice [12]. Nevertheless, the profession is now moving into
more important areas. For instance, the concept of standards of
care is an important issue in which nursing is well ahead of other
disciplines in the health care industry. The vision and foresight
that led to formulation of minimum standards of nursing care
have already had a far-reaching impact on the provision of health
care in this society. As major issues relevant to the delivery of
health care are discussed in the public and political arena, their
impact will become more evident, first because nurses will begin
to recognize that we have a stronger voice in determining the outcome of the decisions, and second because we will have a way of
measuring the effectiveness of the nursing care we provide, thereby
proving its worth to patients and to the health care system.

There have been successful nurse researchers, both in education
and in practice, who have contributed significant research findings
that relate to nursing practice. Among these, the Lysaught report
cites Hoffman and Maislenco for their research relevant to caring
for postpartum patients, Elwood's work with chronic lung disease
and the physiological responses to breathing exercises, Pfandler's
with exercise and its relation to rehabilitation of stroke patients,
Pinneo's study of coronary care and Resnick and Lewis on

286 ambulatory care [12]. These five projects are listed because they are illustrative of the wide range of research possibilities available as well as a demonstration of nurses successfully contributing to the profession through research. The list also points up the fact that success can be achieved, and since "nothing succeeds like success," perhaps it will spur more nurses to become involved in an investigative process to solve some of the problems of nursing practice. Research can also point the way to more effective, efficient and economical use of the available womanpower in nursing. At the same time, nursing will be able to demonstrate that nursing care is an important, successful part of patient care through such criteria as improvement in patient condition; evidence of early, well-planned discharge; a reduced incidence of readmission; and longer periods of stabilized condition. Proof such as these criteria can provide will increase our professional power base in controlling our own practice and in determining the direction the health care industry will go in the future.

I am not suggesting that nursing be entirely responsible for the total health care picture, nor am I suggesting that we want to obtain power in order to dominate the health care industry. We have all seen the consequences of allowing any one branch of a profession involved in health care services to gain total control over the whole. It seems apparent that model is outdated and inefficient in our complex society. What I am advocating is open-mindedness on the part of all health care professionals to new and innovative models based on scientific research carried out by those in our professions who have the capabilities and interests to do so. Recognition of the need for research as well as the outcome of research is vital in the nursing segment of health care services. Until all three aspects of nursing — education, research and practice — begin to work together to achieve research goals, recognition and success for nursing and nurses will remain the oddity they are now. Until those nurses in practice learn to appreciate the efforts of education and research, we will not have many successful practitioners. Until those nurses who are responsible for education pay attention to practitioners and researchers regarding updating curricula, we will not have many successful nurse educators. Until those in research are willing to listen to practitioners and educators regarding what needs to be researched, we will not have many

successful nurse researchers. The intricate balance between
the three areas must be maintained so that each section has its
own autonomy while maintaining the integrity of the whole.
In these concerns, nursing is not unique. Each profession has to
be able to maintain a similar balance between practice, research
and education. It seems to me that those professions that maintain a more equal balance among the three parts are the ones
perceived as being most successful. Are those professions which
are predominantly women's professions less likely to maintain
that intricate balance? And is that secondary to the idea that
women view other women as more of a threat? Or is it because
those professions we see as masculine only *seem* more balanced
because they are perceived as being more prestigious and more
successful?

Occupational success for women has been slow in developing
but seems to be a reachable goal in the foreseeable future. When
the occupation of nursing is viewed by nurses and others as a
successful one, just as medicine, law or engineering is now, there
will be more successful nurses. Epstein speaks of this as the
"charisma of office" [8]. This phenomenon is part of the
reason for the numbers of successful men in science, medicine,
law and management. Women have been denied access to the same
charisma primarily because they have been relegated to professions
and occupations that do not have it. Once nursing is perceived to
be a successful occupation — not just a good work choice for
women — successful nurses will be the rule rather than the exception.
Right now, there are successful nurses on all levels. The *idea* of
successful nurses is still considered odd, however. People do not
define nurses in terms of success. Under the best of circumstances
nurses are defined as being "good" nurses, good being individually
defined by whoever is speaking. More importantly, nurses rarely
define other nurses in terms of being successful.

The whole concept of success is something that women have
been reluctant to attack, fearful of destroying what few strides
forward we have made in our struggle for equality. Throughout
our lives we are encouraged to fail, to avoid success, to be antisuccessful. The idea of achievement in an occupational field of
our choice is incongruous to many of us. In *Women and Success:
The Anatomy of Achievement,* 12 women who are exemplary

figures of success in the sciences give personal accounts of how they believe they achieved success. All 12 believe their professional lives have enhanced their relationships with their husbands and children. These women are unusual in having reached such high levels of success but are *not* unusual in the sense that they are the *only* women who could have done so — given support and encouragement, many women, including nurses, can also achieve success. The circumstances that allowed those women to continue their personal growth and development are varied and range throughout their life from infancy to adulthood. Certainly one of those variables is a husband who supported the wife's need for personal identity and recognition. Bunting says "the search of identity might better be recognized as a search for a meaningful role" [13]. Clearly, this seems to be true in nursing as more and more nurses focus the attention of leaders in the health care system on the aspects of nursing that need attention. Nurses are saying that their role in nursing must be meaningful to them — the individual nurse!

The 12 successful scientists are all married, and so are a great number of nurses. They too need ways of achieving success in their careers and marriages. It is my fervent hope that more nurses who marry will stay in nursing — that they will look for ways to meet their professional identity needs from the leaders in nursing. For a variety of reasons, the nursing profession *needs* more married women who can successfully combine career and marriage. Certainly, we need them as role models for younger women who are contemplating nursing as a career but have ambivalent feelings about being able to keep up with advances in nursing if they decide to marry and/or have children. We also need the married women among them who are successful in nursing because they can be inspirations to *all* women as they find means of meeting their identity and recognition needs. Successful married women in nursing also are needed to decrease the likelihood of discrimination against all women, but particularly against single women. Bunting puts it much more succinctly: "Until it is demonstrated that women with families can contribute effectively in demanding professions, younger women will continue to face cruel decisions and single women to experience senseless discrimination" [13].

How can women with families go about demonstrating that they can contribute effectively in the demanding professions? It seems to me that women who want to demonstrate their effectiveness need to bring about some social change. "In effecting social change one selects the most significant problem that one thinks one can resolve with the skills and resources at one's disposal" [13]. Perhaps in nursing, as in other demanding professions, the most significant social problem we can select is that of the attitudes and behaviors of men. Bearing in mind the theories set forth in previous chapters about planned change, the obvious place to begin may well be with our husbands. Married women who want to achieve success in their chosen field need to learn how to use both power strategy and attitude change strategy on their husbands as well as men from whom they seek employment and with whom they work. The intent is to raise the consciousness level of these men to the idea that married women have needs for identity and recognition that are best met through success in their occupation or profession. In Caroline Bird's book *What Every Woman Needs To Know To Get Paid What She's Worth,* the question is asked: "Does it pay to go back to college or graduate school to start a new career?" Ms. Bird uses Florence Gaynor's success story to prove that it is best to have a specific goal in mind.* Effective behavior change always involves some manipulation and control, according to Kelman [14]. Women have long been accused, rightly or wrongly, of using manipulation to gain their ends. Raising the consciousness of husbands seems to be one of the "right" times to use it. I would hope that there are more than 12 husbands willing and able to support and encourage their wives to achieve as much success as those in *Women and Success.* Women should not passively wait for enlightenment to come to men, however; they should actively pursue ways of bringing insight to their husbands. Sometimes insight is gained through very mundane facts. For example, "in March 1969 over half of all American families depended on two incomes, and the 'extra' working member was far more apt to be the wife than to be the son or daughter of the principal breadwinner" [15].

*At age 40 Ms. Gaynor went back to school for a master's degree in public health administration. After graduating through a succession of several jobs, she became the first woman to be appointed administrator of the New Jersey Medical School College of Medicine and Dentistry and the largest hospital in New Jersey.

290 The argument that a family can live better with two salaries than one is powerful even for the most recalcitrant spouse in these days of recession and inflation.

My life experiences are similar, in many instances, to those of the 12 successful women. I chose nursing because it offered a marketable skill — one I felt I could use in a variety of ways and places. It also seemed to offer a professional career in which I could meet my own needs for recognition and identity, earn money by my efforts and choose a variety of settings in which to practice. I was 28 years old with no previous college education when I enrolled in a baccalaureate degree program. I had been married 11 years to a bricklayer with no formal education past high school and was the mother of three daughters aged 4 through 10. We had a comfortable home, friends and other accoutrements of lower-middle-class people in a small town. In other words, by the standards of many people I should have been content. And in many ways I was. But I realized that I could never really be satisfied until I proved to myself that there was more to my identity as a person than to be someone's wife or someone's mother. There was also a very real need to earn money, not only because we needed it then, but also to have a way to support myself and my children if my husband should die or become disabled — a very real possibility in construction work. Ten years later I have a master's degree and know I could be well into a doctoral program if I desired. I managed to commute 60 miles a day, run a home with minimal outside help (a babysitter for our youngest child), work part-time while an undergraduate and full-time as a graduate student, have another baby and maintain good enough grades to be an honor student and graduate in the upper third of my class. Did it bring ruin to my children, lower my husband's self-esteem or destroy our marriage? Absolutely not! Just as with the women in *Women and Success,* it has enhanced my relationships with both my husband and my children. My children see me as a successful woman who is a nurse and their mother, just as they see their father as a successful man who is a mason and their father. They are highly independent, intelligent, aggressive young women who have a well-rounded, beautiful concept of themselves. They can clearly perceive their future roles as women who can combine motherhood, marriage and career. They can also see themselves as single women whose needs for personal recognition and identity can be met through means other than marriage and motherhood.

Did I effect any social change? I believe so, if one takes into consideration that the social change that occurred was in the attitudes and behaviors of a very small group — my husband, my children and a few friends. Because I pursued a desire to meet my own needs for recognition and identity as an individual person and not just as someone's mother or someone's wife, I raised one man's level of awareness concerning women and four daughters' consciousness that women are capable of intellectually pursuing and gaining a goal. Convincing my husband that my education could be the best insurance policy he ever bought was possibly the most significant problem I resolved with the skills and resources at my disposal.

John Gardner once said, "A society gets the kind of excellence it values." If a society such as the health care system really *values* excellence in the field of nursing, it should be willing to start to explore ways in which excellence can be encouraged, nourished and allowed to grow, particularly where women are concerned. There should be more than the one way I chose for women to achieve success and excellence in such an essential service as health care. The Radcliffe Institute has "set up fellowship programs to assist mature women with children who wish to continue advanced studies on a part-time schedule and who need financial assistance to do so" [13]. All the women they have assisted have continued their chosen profession. This is a magnificent success story and one that the health care industry should be cognizant of. There are a variety of ways it could be adapted to meet the needs of nurses and the health care system. For instance, a nurse with a baccalaureate degree who chose to stay home while her children were young could use such a system to work on an advanced degree, to keep abreast of new technologies and advances in nursing or to do independent study concerning some aspect of nursing that she did not have time to study while working full-time. When her children reached school age, she could again enter the active field of nursing without having lost ground in her area of expertise, be a better prepared nurse (thereby increasing her dollar value to herself and her employer) and perhaps have new solutions to problems in nursing care that she had researched.

How could such a system be instituted so that nurses could use it and so that standards of excellence could be maintained? The suggestions that follow are certainly not in-depth analyses of the problem, but they are food for thought concerning ways such a program *might* be started. It seems to me that we already have what could well be the catalyst for such a program, and that is Comprehensive Health Care Planning Agencies. They already review and recommend plans for health care agencies and funds for research, health care personnel needs, educational needs and other aspects of the health care industry. Perhaps it is plausible for Comprehensive Health Care Planning Agencies to be involved with universities and colleges in developing programs such as Radcliffe's. How the program would be disseminated throughout a Comprehensive Health Planning region might create some difficulties, but they should not be insurmountable and might depend on the need for the program and the distribution of people in any one planning region. Faculty members of colleges and universities could be used as advisors to individual students or to groups of students. This aspect would have advantages for both the students and the faculty members, as it would increase faculty's involvement in a larger community and decrease the isolation so prevalent in nursing while giving students opportunities to utilize role-models with greater expertise than their own. I realize that such an endeavor would be expensive, but when one considers that educated women — and this includes nurses — represent an enormous economic opportunity for this country, the expense involved seems worthwhile. "There are 5½ million college graduates and 8 million women with some college training in America today. Women represent 38 percent of *all* college graduates and 34 percent of all graduate students. The current waste of talent in American women cannot be allowed to continue. Given the necessary capital and a marketable product or service, a business needs an able and productive staff and a maximum demand for its product or service. The educated working family woman provides both" [16]. If the current waste is not to continue, we must find ways to keep educated women in the working world or in fields such as research that will benefit their working world. Programs such as Radcliffe's seem to be one answer for nursing's educated women.

Another way such a program might be funded is through the

already established Professional Nurse Traineeship Program.
Originally established in 1956, it has been continued and expanded through federal legislation. "From fiscal year 1957 to fiscal year 1972, 33,989 long-term traineeships were awarded to increase the supply of registered nurses prepared for teaching, administration and supervision" [9]. Needless to say, it would have to be greatly extended and expanded in order to fulfill the need, but in the long run perhaps it would be less expensive than the continual loss of educated nurses who leave practice to have children and never return because they are too far behind the advances that have been made in their field. Perhaps it would be less expensive than educating nurses to teach, only to discover they are behind their students in new ideas because they lack the time and money to stop teaching in order to do in-depth research into nursing education. Perhaps it would be less expensive than the poor quality of care many consumers receive because nurses refuse to return to nursing for lack of job enrichment, educational advancement or professional growth. "In fiscal year 1972 the nation spent 83.4 billion dollars on health, according to Social Security Administration estimates. This represents 7.6 percent of the country's total gross national product. Although the private sector was the major source of funds for health care expenditures, twenty-five percent of the total came from federal funds and 12 percent from state and local governments" [9]. It seems to me that the consumer, the federal government and state and local governments should be interested in getting the greatest possible value for their dollars, and that might well be accomplished through assuring nurses and other health care personnel of adequate continuing education that would keep them in the mainstream of providing care, or at least give them an adequate means of returning to it. A system such as this would enhance the excellence that society values because it would be a higher order of excellence. One of the reasons women are so frequently put down by the sexist society we live in is because it is said we do not excel. We quit, drop out, refuse to commit ourselves wholeheartedly to our careers — at least by men's standards. Ms. Bunting's concepts are very concrete methods of raising the expectations of excellence for women in our society. When men and women can see that excellence is just as apt to be a part of woman's behavior as it is man's, excellence may well be rewarded

294 on an equal basis. Society and the economy suffer along with the health care industry when professional nurses are not provided adequate justification for putting their education to work.

Another, perhaps more subtle aspect is that many young women feel they can either have a marriage/motherhood career *or* a professional career, but not both. Because young women cannot see a solution to this dilemma and because they realize that the family has become so small that it is not an adequate focus for a full-time, life-time commitment, they opt for a professional career. Obviously, this is a threat to the family unit as we know it in this society. The answer seems to lie in the ability of men (who control all the major institutions in our society) to change their attitudes, values and behaviors. Women will have to realize that "discrimination against women — the requirement that they be single women or single-minded super-women in order to have a career — will not end until women have the option to embark on careers before the birth of their children, contract their commitment when their children are small, and expand it as family responsibilities diminish" [13]. Sociologists Orden and Bradburn claim that "a woman's freedom to choose among alternative life styles is an important predictor of happiness in marriage" [17]. Freedom of choice also involves freedom to change. This obvious point has significant inferences for nurses, because freedom to change is "freedom to break up a situation that has hardened into discomfort" [17]. Surely most nurses will agree that our situation has indeed hardened into discomfort.

Change is never easy and sometimes it is traumatic and occasionally useless. In some cases (nursing for instance), it can bring imagination and creativity to bear on old, stereotyped, outdated ideas and begin the development of new solutions that will extend beyond the new aspects of the situation.

It is past time for nursing to use freedom of choice, however limited, to open the doors of nursing and the minds of nurses to new and imaginative ideas and solutions. When this occurs, nursing will indeed have become a successful profession and nurses will be recognized as successful people.

1. Viscott, David. Nineteen Ways to Be Uniquely Yourself. *New Woman*, Vol. 5, No. 5, September—October 1975.
2. Kundsin, Ruth B. To Autonomous Women: An Introduction. In *Women and Success: The Anatomy of Achievement*, Kundsin, Ruth B. (Ed.). New York: William Morrow, 1974.
3. Maslow, Abraham. *Toward a Psychology of Being*, 2nd ed. New York: Van Nostrand, 1968.
4. Komisor, Lucy. The Image of Women in Advertising. In *Woman in Sexist Society: Studies in Power and Powerlessness*, Gornick, Vivian, and Moran, Barbara (Eds.). New York: Basic Books, 1971.
5. Viscott, David. If You're Dissatisfied with Your Life. *New Woman*, Vol. 5, No. 5, September—October 1975.
6. Sex Role Dissonance. *Human Behavior*, Vol. 4, No. 9, September 1975.
7. Robertson, Wyndham. The Highest Ranking Women in Big Business. *Fortune*, Vol. 87, No. 4, April 1973.
8. Epstein, Cynthia Fuchs. Bringing Women In: Rewards, Punishments, and the Structure of Achievement. In *Women and Success: The Anatomy of Achievement*, Kundsin, Ruth B. (Ed.). New York: William Morrow, 1974.
9. *Facts about Nursing 72—73*. Kansas City, Mo: American Nurses' Association, 1974.
10. Poirier, Brooke. Loeb Center: What Nursing Can — and Should — Be. *The American Nurse*, Vol. 7, No. 1, January 1975.
11. Lambertson, Eleanor. The Changing Role of Nursing and Its Regulation. *Nursing Clinics of North America*, Vol. 9, No. 3, September 1974.
12. Lysaught, Jerome P. *An Abstract for Action*. New York: Blakiston Div., McGraw-Hill, 1970.
13. Bunting, Mary I. Education: A Nurturant if not a Determinant of Professional Success. In *Women and Success: The Anatomy of Achievement*, Kundsin, Ruth B. (Ed.). New York: William Morrow, 1974.
14. Kelman, Herbert. Manipulation of Human Behavior: An Ethical Dilemma for the Social Scientist. In *The Planning of Change*, Bennis, Warren, Benne, Kenneth, and Chin, Robert (Eds.). New York: Holt, Rinehart and Winston, 1969.
15. Janeway, Elizabeth. *Man's World, Woman's Place: A Study in Social Mythology*. New York: Dell, 1971.
16. Swartz, Felice N. Women and Employers: Their Related Needs and Attitudes. In *Women and Success: The Anatomy of Achievement*, Kundsin, Ruth B. (Ed.). New York: William Morrow, 1974.
17. Orden, Susan, and Bradburn, Norman. Working Wives and Family Happiness. *American Journal of Sociology*, Vol. 74, No. 4, January 1969.

11   In Process

Marlene Grissum and Carol Spengler

We are in process, *continually evolving,*
and we will no longer be made to
feel inferior or ineffective for knowing
and being what we are at any given
moment [1].
Robin Morgan

Throughout this book, we have been discussing issues and problems of nurses and of women at large. These issues are charged with emotion, but we have attempted to see through the emotionalism and present some rational answers.

The socialization of women is one of these issues. Certainly, all of us, men and women, go through a process of socialization as we progress from infancy to adulthood. However, up to now, men have set the tone for the socialization of both sexes. It is now past time for women and men to begin thinking in terms of what human characteristics we want to inculcate into future generations — not what is masculine or what is feminine, but rather what is individually human. It is time for parents to start stressing the individual child's uniqueness — not because that child happens to be male or female — but because there is no other person exactly like that particular child. Robin Morgan declares "there is a difference between individualism and individuality — and . . . the latter is precious and to be cherished" [1]. The quality that distinguishes one person from another (individuality) will lead us

298 away from socializing *all* females to be passive, submissive and dependent and *all* males to be aggressive, dominant and independent. Our world needs men and women with both "masculine" and "feminine" characteristics — it needs people who are oriented toward those aspects of our society that are *humane* rather than either masculine or feminine. We are rapidly approaching a time when parents will view their responsibility for socialization in terms of human sexuality rather than gender sexuality. When this process reaches the point where it is synthesis rather than antithesis, we will have overcome one of our major barriers to an egalitarian society.

Another area that is highly charged with emotion is our sense of self-love or self-esteem. As we are socialized to become a part of the society in which we live, we are also taught a sense of our own worth. In the past, women have been taught to believe that we are worth less than others — our sense of worthlessness destroys our self-love — and our self-esteem has remained microscopic in comparison to men's sense of self-worth and self-esteem. We have attempted throughout this book to point out ways women can increase their sense of worth. Certainly a part of this process includes the socialization of women to believe in themselves — to be aware of themselves as persons with rights and privileges like other persons. It is difficult to increase our sense of self-esteem if we are not aware that we have been socialized to believe that we are not valued as much as men are by our society. As we raise our level of awareness, we become cognizant of the fact that we have been exploited and oppressed longer than any other group [1]. Once we have reached that state of awareness, we can then take action to increase our sense of *self*-worth. After all, until we believe we have value, it is not likely that others will. Once we begin to love and value ourselves, we will develop the ability to become winners. We will be able to recognize our own uniqueness, reveal our real selves rather than stereotypic images, become authentic people and be comfortable with that authenticity and reality. With the comfortableness comes the realization that we are no longer powerless.

The idea that women are powerless or powerful is based on sociological myths and therefore is based on emotionalism. Whether one views women as powerless or powerful probably depends on whether one is a man or a woman. Both views are mythical in origin, however, and both are actually perpetuated by the mythmakers in our society. As we have pointed out, myths are based on emotion and cannot be disproved by fact or logic alone. In order to disprove the myth of female power or female powerlessness, we must seek answers "in reality to meet those needs which the myth answers in fantasy" [2]. The fact is that women are neither powerful nor powerless. Until we women learn how to use the potential power we have, however, it will appear to others as if we are powerless. We can also anticipate that when we learn to use our potential resources to exert our power, others, primarily men, will perceive us as a threat. Once more, the mythical ghost of female power, with its ability to dominate men, will exert a strong influence on male behavior. The emotion predominantly involved is fear — "the mythic fear that sees change as destruction" [2]. Nevertheless, it is time for our society to move out of our mythical past and into the realistic present. Both men and women who are threatened by the realities of female power will have opportunities to become aware that women can and will use power to institute constructive, positive changes in our society.

The whole concept of change is another area fraught with emotion. Most people are resistant to change on one level or another. When a large segment of the population of women start instituting and demanding changes in our societal behavior and *mores,* however, many women and most men begin to feel threatened. "For if the female role is changing, men's role has got to take account of the change and adapt to it, so men feel the pressure to change, too, a pressure which they did not inaugurate and must consequently, predictably, resent" [2]. But, resented or not, feared or welcomed, change has become an integral part of our society, and all of us will have to learn how to accept it into our lives with ever-increasing rapidity and regularity. How women accept it and learn to use the strategies connected with it will, in great measure, determine our sense of self-esteem, our power and our control over our own lives. Throughout this book we have attempted to demonstrate ways that women (and nurses) can begin to inaugurate affirmative action to develop equal opportunities for women.

When a specific group of people in society come to realize that

300 they are not receiving a fair share of the benefits and rewards of that society, social conflicts develop. This conflict may give birth to a movement that catches on and grows to such major proportions that it touches the lives of great numbers of people. It may eventually lead to social reforms of such magnitude that the changes become incorporated and institutionalized into society. Once these reforms are institutionalized and remain over time, society tends to adapt to them and eventually to look upon them as having always existed. The reforms then become the accepted customs and *mores* of the time. The rights, privileges and rewards enjoyed by many Americans today are largely taken for granted. When we read about our ancestors and our early history, we are grateful to those who struggled to establish our country as a democracy. Except for those who are serious and continuous students of American history, however, most Americans do not spend a great deal of time thinking about our heritage and the way things were in the past. Most people are more concerned with the present and the future. Our greatest dream is to live to see the day when equality will exist for women in all areas of society — politically, economically, socially and psychologically. The day when women are truly free to make choices without sexist barriers and are respected for those choices, regardless of what they are, is a dream in the making. It is exciting to envision the time when women will have the same opportunities as men to develop their potential in whatever areas they choose. Even more exciting is the idea that this condition will exist as an established custom and will be taken for granted as an acceptable social norm. To think ahead to the time in the future when we, as women, will be legitimatized as full, contributing, respected and valued members of society is a heady thought. For those who are skeptical that this will ever happen, we suggest a review of social reform in the past as well as an evaluation of present efforts to bring about social changes in relation to women. We are happy to report, in case anyone is doubtful, that the women's movement in this country is alive and well. It is not only very much alive, but it is growing, maturing, surviving and succeeding.

Jo Freeman, a political scientist, has studied the origins of the women's liberation movement extensively. She states that social movement can "be conceived of as having a center and a periphery"

An investigation into a movement's origins must be made in order for a group to constitute a social movement that is capable of bringing about significant changes. These propositions are as follows: (1) a primary prerequisite for spontaneous activity is the need for a preexisting communication network or infrastructure within the social base of a movement. This communication system helps a group to spread the word regarding their concerns. Without it, the protest does not become generalized and soon dissolves; (2) the communications network must be one that is co-optable (chosen by joint action) to the new ideas of the beginning movement; therefore, it must be composed of like-minded people who have similar backgrounds, experience or locations in relation to the social structure; (3) from this emerge two distinct patterns that may overlap. In the first, a crisis stimulates the network into some form of spontaneous action in a new direction. In the second, people begin disseminating a new idea or begin organizing a new type of organization [3]. As diverse as the women's concerns, styles of living and ways of organizing have been in the movement, it is easy to see that these propositions have been met. This explains why the women's movement has emerged as a significant social movement that is responsible for some of the long-overdue reforms that are beginning to take place.

If we consider the nursing profession in light of these three important propositions, it could be said that we have all the requisites necessary for the development of a significant social movement that could lead to important reforms and improvements within the health care system. Nurses already have a viable communications network within the profession. In all that has been pointed out in this book, it should be clear that there is a crisis in nursing and a crisis in the health care system. All we need to do now is to generalize our protest, disseminate our ideas and organize our efforts in collective activities. The outcome could be the transformation of an inadequate, inefficient health care system into one that is capable of delivering effective and humane service to the American public.

Will nurses be in the vanguard of this crucial social movement?

1. Morgan, Robin. Rights of Passage. *Ms.,* Vol. 4, No. 3, September 1975, p. 98.
2. Janeway, Elizabeth. *Man's World, Woman's Place: A Study in Social Mythology.* New York: Dell, 1971.
3. Freeman, Jo. The Origins of the Women's Liberation Movement. In *Changing Women in a Changing Society,* Huber, Joan (Ed.). Chicago: University of Chicago Press, 1973.

Index